£19.95

LANCHEST

Mu

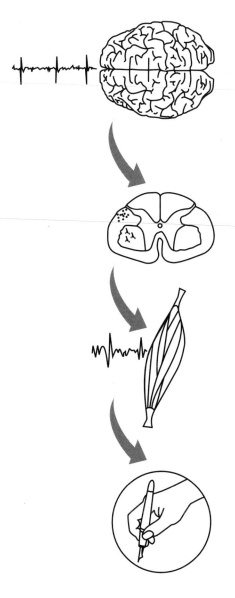

Neural Control
of Skilled Human
Movement

Editor
F.W.J. Cody

PORTLAND PRESS

Published by Portland Press Ltd., 59 Portland Place,
London W1N 3AJ, U.K.
on behalf of the Physiological Society

In North America orders should be sent to Ashgate Publishing Co.,
Old Post Road, Brookfield, VT 05036-9704, U.S.A.

ISBN 1 85578 081 X   ISSN 0969-8116

Coventry University

British Library Cataloguing in Publication Data
A catalogue record for this book is available from
the British Library

Cover illustration by T. Beer
Book design by A. Moyes

Typeset by Portland Press Ltd.
and printed in Great Britain by Henry Ling Ltd., Dorchester

P06623

Contents

Preface

Movements make man. Uniquely, we can write and talk. Our everyday lives depend on precise control of the muscles that produce finger movements and speech sounds. A healthy student takes such highly skilled movements for granted, they seem easy. Yet how difficult it is for his/her teacher to explain how the nervous system manages the task.

This volume arose out of an enjoyable and thought-provoking Teaching Symposium which was held at Manchester University and supported by the Physiological Society. The topic of movement control has always been notoriously difficult for students and a particular challenge to their teachers. The mechanisms can be taught with confidence, but it is far harder to convey a sense of function. Hence, having assimilated a wealth of information about cerebellar pathways, circuitry and neuro-transmitters, students are still left asking the question, 'What does the cerebellum actually do?'.

A major aim of this volume was to consider such basic questions and adopt a functional approach.

The book focuses on skilled movements in man, while drawing upon vital evidence obtained in other species. Attention is mainly directed at movements of the hand and arm, which have been studied most fully. The production of speech sounds is considered to be another important example of skilled movement. Concise up-dates of current understanding of the roles of the main motor centres — cerebral cortex, basal ganglia, cerebellum and spinal cord — in skilled movement and its clinical impairments, are provided by a group of neuroscientists renowned for their research expertise and enthusiasm for teaching.

Frederick W. J. Cody
Manchester, 1995

Abbreviations

BP	Bereitschaftspotential
CM	cortico-motoneuronal
CNS	central nervous system
CS	corticoid stimulus
1DI	first dorsal interosseous
Del	deltoid
EDC	extensor digitorum communis
EEG	electroencephalograph
EMG	electromyograph
EPSP	excitatory post-synaptic potential
F_O	fundamental frequency
GABA	γ-amino butyric acid
GPe	globus pallidus, external segment
GPi	globus pallidus, internal segment
GTO	Golgi tendon organ
HVC	high vocal centre
IO	inferior olive
LCST	lateral corticospinal tract
LIP	intraparietal sulcus
LTD	long-term depression
LTP	long-term potentiation
MI	primary motor cortex
MPTP	N-methyl-4-phenyl-1,2,3,6 tetrahydropyridine
MRP	movement-related potential
NA	nucleus ambiguus
NMR	nictitating membrane reflex
PAG	periaqueductal gray
P cell	Purkinje cell
PET	positron emission tomography
PMC	premotor cortex
PPC	posterior parietal cortex
PSF	post-spike facilitation
PTN	pyrimidal tract neuron
RA	robust nucleus of the archistriatum
RIFM	relatively independent finger movement
SMA	supplementary motor area
SNpc	substantia nigra pars compacta
SNpr	substantia nigra pars reticulata
STA	spike-triggered averaging
TMS	transcranial magnetic stimulation
VL	ventralis lateratis
VOR	vestibulo-ocular reflex

Cortical control of skilled movements

Roger. N. Lemon

Sobell Department of Neurophysiology, Institute of Neurology, London WC1N 3BG, U.K.

Introduction

In man the primary motor area (Brodmann's area 4, or MI) of the cerebral cortex plays a major role in the control of normal voluntary movements. It communicates with all the brainstem and spinal centres necessary for the execution of these movements. It also represents the main means through which other important motor structures, including the cerebellum and basal ganglia, gain access to these centres. Although considerable recovery is often seen following stroke affecting the motor cortex or its descending pathways, many patients are left with one of its most debilitating effects: the permanent loss of skilled hand and finger movements. Essential everyday movements such as writing, doing up buttons, or handling a knife and fork are difficult or impossible to perform.

In this chapter, the experimental evidence suggesting a unique role for the corticomotoneuronal (CM) projection in the execution of skilled hand movements will be reviewed. This projection is made up of corticospinal fibres having direct, monosynaptic connections with spinal motoneurons, and particularly with those motoneurons supplying the muscles which move the fingers. In man, the projection also supplies motoneurons of the more proximal muscles acting at the elbow and shoulder. Both 'slow'- and 'fast'-conducting fibres contribute CM synapses. The CM projection is excitatory and found only in primates, and there is a close correspondence between the degree of digital dexterity and the number of CM projections.

I shall then consider how the CM system contributes to skilled movements, and the importance of sensory feedback for both motor control and the activity of CM cells. Finally I shall discuss how the CM system is organized at the cortical level.

▶ How does a voluntary movement come about? One model envisages three stages for this process. The 'plan' of the movement describes its objective or goal; the 'program' has to translate that plan and work out the necessary movements (kinematics) and forces (dynamics) that will be needed to implement it, leading to the execution of the movement.

The neural substrate for skilled hand movements

Skilled hand movements are an essential part of our culture: our technology, communication, art and science depend upon them. The complex skeleto-muscular apparatus of the hand is managed by a distributed central motor system. This has been elegantly revealed by recent positron emission tomography (PET) studies showing that many different areas of the brain, including the sensorimotor and premotor cortex, supplementary motor area (SMA), posterior parietal cortex, basal ganglia and cerebellum are active during performance of a learned task. How do all these structures contribute to the movement, and do their contributions differ?

One model of movement control suggests a serial process in which the starting point is a 'plan', describing the goal or objective of the movement. In this model the plan of the movement is independent of the skeleto-muscular system needed to produce the movement. An example might be the writing of a signature: this looks very similar whether it is written with the dominant hand, non-dominant hand, mouth or foot [1].

The plan is then processed to form a 'program', containing a description of the way in which the plan is to be implemented: for example, which segments of which limb are to be involved. The capacity to perform a given task in a variety of ways is referred to as 'motor equivalence' [1] and it reflects the many degrees of freedom of a multiarticulate limb. But the number of possible ways in which one can, for example, reach out and grasp an object, is very large indeed. An important issue in motor control is just how the brain solves this 'degrees of freedom' problem. How does it select a particular set of joint angles and joint torques to produce the required movement? Part of the solution may rest in relatively 'hard-wired' functional synergies involving small groups of muscles.

In the final stage of the process, the 'execution' of the movement, the appropriate groups of muscles are contracted leading to changes in forces and torques, acting at different joints, to produce the required movement.

While this model has some attractive features, the implementation of these different stages in discrete neural structures has been challenged [2]. Although neurons in a given part of the motor system encode different properties of the movement (e.g. force or direction), the encoding is not discrete. The population of neurons within a single region may encode several different functions. Finally, there is a considerable overlap in the timing of neuronal activity in different structures. This argues against a simple serial process such as that described above. It has long been known that the central nervous system (CNS) becomes active well in advance of the first signs of muscular activity. Even in the motor cortex, with direct influence over the motoneurons involving short central delays in the order of a few milliseconds, many neurons become active up to 100 ms before movement. These delays are long enough to allow information, related to the different stages of movement production, to pass several times through cortico-basal ganglia and cortico-cerebellar loops before the movement actually begins. These loops are re-entrant in nature: projections from motor cortex to both the basal ganglia and cerebellum influence pathways projecting back to the cortex. Thus more recent work suggests that the different elements contributing to the movement: plan, program and execution, are processed in parallel [2].

Just as the emphasis has moved from serial to parallel models of movement control, so has increased attention been given to the parallel routes through which the cerebral cortex can control movement. Access to the final common path, the motoneurons and muscles, from key motor structures including the neostriatum, lateral cerebellum and association cortex are largely relayed through the motor areas of the cerebral cortex. These areas give rise to descending pathways which influence the spinal machinery for movement either directly, via the corticospinal tract, or indirectly via projections to midbrain and brainstem centres which themselves give rise to descending pathways, such as the rubrospinal, reticulospinal and vestibulospinal tracts. Recent investigations [3] have demonstrated that the primary motor cortex probably accounts for only about half of the corticospinal fibres originating in the frontal lobe. Other important areas giving rise to the corticospinal tract include the premotor, SMA, and cingulate motor areas. Each of these areas projects to the primary motor cortex, but can also influence the spinal cord through its corticospinal projections. However, the contrasting properties of neurons in these different areas suggest that their contribution is not simply a parallel output nor indeed a redundant one.

CM projections and relatively independent finger movements (RIFM)

Present evidence suggests that the CM projection is mainly derived from the caudal part of the primary motor cortex. A large number of electrophysiological, anatomical and behavioural studies (reviewed in [4]) have supported the view that this projection provides the capacity for the performance of RIFM.

First, the CM system has long been known to exert particularly strong effects on the motoneurons of muscles acting on the hand and fingers. This finding has been amply confirmed in man by the use of transcranial magnetic stimulation (TMS) of the motor cortex. TMS can directly excite the cells of origin of the corticospinal tract and this results in short-latency electromyographic (EMG) responses in upper-limb muscles. The form and time course of these responses suggest they are mediated by the CM system. The largest responses to TMS are generally found in the most distal muscles, i.e. the hand muscles [4,5]. All CM connections appear to be excitatory; inhibition was shown to take place through disynaptic pathways via spinal interneurons.

Secondly, there is a general correspondence between the degree of digital dexterity and the existence of direct CM projections. As shown in Fig. 1, such projections are sparse or absent in non-primates, which have little or no capacity for independent digit movement. In the macaque (Old World) monkey, the CM projection is limited to the most dorso-lateral parts of the motoneuronal cell groups of lamina IX, where the motoneurons supplying the hand and finger muscles are located [6]. RIFM are

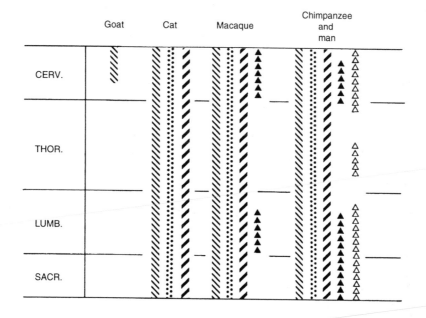

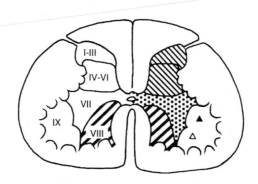

Fig. I. Schematic diagram illustrating the termination of corticospinal fibres in four different representative species: goat, cat, macaque monkey and chimpanzee/man

The upper diagram indicates the spinal level (cervical to sacral) reached by projections to different parts of the spinal grey matter, as shown in the section below. The symbols represent terminations: in the dorsal horn (laminae I–III and IV–VI, thin hatching); in lamina VII (dots) and VIII (thick hatching) of the intermediate zone; and CM projections to lamina IX (triangles). Note the bilateral projection to lamina VIII, the absence of CM projections in the cat and goat, and the presence, in chimpanzee and man of CM projections, to both dorsolateral motoneurons innervating muscles of the extremity (filled triangles) and to ventromedial motoneurons of the axial and truncal muscles (open triangles). Adapted from ref. [6].

best developed in the great apes and in man: these species have extensive CM connections, still heaviest and most numerous to the muscles of the hand, but including projections to all proximal muscles of the upper limb (open triangles in Fig. 1).

Thirdly, in young primates, the development of RIFM and the maturation of direct CM connections appear to occur in parallel. Newborn human or macaque infants exhibit little capacity for skilled hand control. For the infant macaque the most notable feature is a powerful grasp which ensures that it does not lose hold of its mother as she travels around. Lawrence and Hopkins showed that infant monkeys did not exhibit RIFM until around 3 months of age, and that a mature pattern of RIFM was not seen until 7–8 months (see [4,7]). Anatomical studies show that the newborn monkey possesses few, if any, direct CM projections, but that they are present by around 6 months of age.

This last result has been confirmed by using TMS. The short-latency responses evoked by TMS in the adult were not found in the newborn monkey, and mature responses did not appear until around 6–8 months of age ([4]; see Fig. 2). The development of functional CM synapses is coupled to an increase in corticospinal tract conduction velocity. However, a functional link between these changes in CM connectivity and the maturation of skilled hand movements is yet to be proven.

Further evidence has come from lesion work: in adult monkeys complete bilateral section of the pyramidal tract permanently abolishes RIFM and similar lesions in newborn monkeys prevent the development of RIFM [7]. The motor deficits resulting from motor cortex lesions in man appear to be due to the loss of the patterned input to the motoneuron plus a loss of the background excitatory drive to the motoneurons, resulting, respectively, in a poverty and weakness of skilled movement.

Although the evidence is that CM projections provide the basic capacity for skilled hand and finger movements, the precise patterning and timing of activity within the tract is determined by other parts of the motor system which themselves ultimately influence the cells of origin of the corticospinal tract. The evolution of a motor skill involves a steady improvement in the employment of this output pathway. The existence of the pathway alone does

not provide for normal voluntary movement, as is shown by the fact that patients with severe motor disorders can have intact conduction within the corticospinal tract [7].

▶ Four lines of evidence suggest that digital dexterity requires the integrity of direct CM connections: (i) these connections have their strongest influence over hand muscles; (ii) there is a good correlation between the digital dexterity of different species and the number of CM connections; (iii) during development there appears to be a parallel maturation of CM connections and skilled finger movements; and (iv) interruption of the descending tracts carrying the CM fibres results in a permanent loss of fine finger movements.

Features of the CM system which contribute to the control of skilled hand movements

What properties of the CM system would allow it to contribute to the execution of skilled independent finger movements? While stimulation studies help us to test for connectivity, they can tell us little about how such connections are employed in natural voluntary movement. It has been essential to adopt a macaque monkey model for studying the function of individual CM cells. This is an appropriate model: the macaque hand is similar to that of man, as is, on present evidence, the neural substrate for its control.

Our approach has been to train macaque monkeys to perform a precision grip task, using the thumb and index finger (see Fig. 3a): the monkey is rewarded for performance of RIFM. After around 3 months of training, the monkey is prepared, under deep general anaesthesia, for recording single cells from the motor cortex contralateral to the trained hand. During this operation two fine stimulating electrodes are implanted within the medullary pyramidal tract. The monkey then receives a full postoperative programme of analgesia and other medication.

CM cells are identified in the conscious monkey using the spike-triggered averaging (STA) method [4,7,8]. This method is illustrated in Fig. 3(a): if a monosynaptic CM connection existed between the pyramidal tract

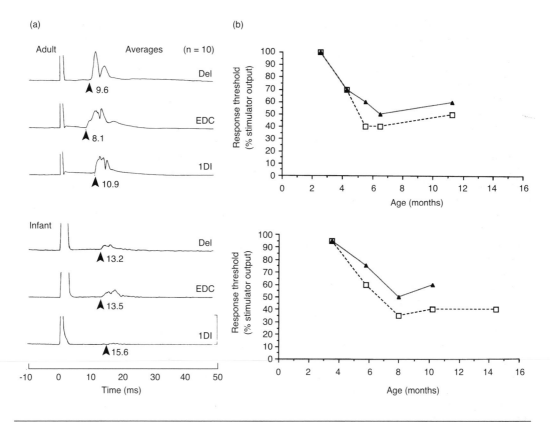

Fig. 2. (a) Comparison of the EMG responses from different muscles to non-invasive magnetic stimulation of the brain in an adult (above) and in an infant monkey aged 2.5 months (below) and (b) longitudinal studies of threshold changes for EMG responses recorded from 1DI following brain stimulation in two infant macaque monkeys under ketamine sedation

(a) Magnetic stimuli were delivered during periods of spontaneous EMG activity recorded during sedation with ketamine. Onset latencies (in ms) of responses are arrowed. In the infant average responses were small and had long latencies in deltoid (Del) and in extensor digitorum communis (EDC); a very small, late response was recorded from the first dorsal interosseous (1DI).

(b) Before 5 months of age the thresholds were high and similar for responses evoked during periods of spontaneous EMG activity (□, active) or quiescence (▲, relaxed); after this age thresholds fell rapidly and were 10–20% lower when there was spontaneous activity. Reproduced with permission from [4].

neuron (PTN) and the motoneuron, the excitatory post-synaptic potentials (EPSPs) produced in the motoneuron by impulses in the PTN should raise its firing probability and some of these EPSPs should actually cause the motoneuron to fire. If a sufficiently large number of motoneuronal discharges occur in response to the CM spikes, then this results in a post-spike facilitation (PSF) of rectified EMG activity, which is revealed in the average as a transient increase in EMG activity time-locked to the

discharge of the CM cell. The evidence that this PSF does indeed represent CM action is reviewed elsewhere [7,8].

The first important feature of the CM system is its direct and powerful influence over the motoneurons supplying the muscles moving the hand and digits. In the example shown in Fig. 4(b), the peak PSF amplitude represents a 38% modulation of the background EMG activity. This direct access bypasses the reflex mechanisms controlling the same motoneurons.

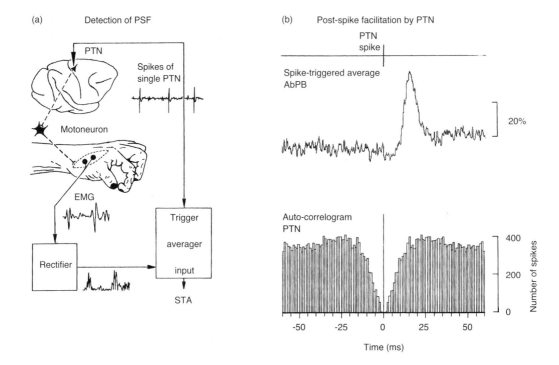

Fig. 3. (a) The use of spike-triggered averaging to detect post-spike facilitation (PSF) of EMG activity recorded from monkey hand muscles and (b) an example of PSF produced in spike-triggered average (STA) of EMG response from a thumb muscle (AbPB) by 9000 PTN spikes

(a) The experimental arrangement is illustrated and the putative CM connection from a single pyramidal tract neuron (PTN) to the motoneurons of the muscle indicated by a broken line. EMG activity is rectified and averaged with respect to PTN spikes. (b) Vertical scale indicates 20% modulation of background EMG level. PTN discharge is at time zero. Auto-correlogram of the PTN spikes is shown below. Reproduced with permission from [4].

For hand-muscle motoneurons these reflex segmental influences are considerably weaker than those acting on motoneurons of more proximal muscles. The spinal component of the stretch reflex is less pronounced, and recurrent (Renshaw) inhibition is weak or absent. The CM system in primates is important because it provides for fractionation of activity within the motoneuron pools to a degree that is not provided by spinal reflex mechanisms; the CM system also permits greater pools to a degree that is not provided by spinal reflex flexibility in the co-activation of small groups of muscles. It must not be forgotten, however, that the densest termination of the corticospinal tract is among the spinal interneurons lying in the intermediate zone of the spinal grey matter, allowing the cortex to participate in the control of spinal reflex mechanisms.

A role in fractionation of muscle activity is further suggested by two other features of the CM projection. CM cells generally influence activity in a small group of target muscles, and these muscles are often active as functional synergists. The divergent influence of a single CM cell can be demonstrated in spike-triggered averages of EMG activity recorded from several different hand and forearm muscles and averaged with respect to spikes from a single CM cell [7,8]. The most reasonable explanation of this result is that the axon of each CM cell diverges to make contact with the motor columns of different muscles, as illustrated schematically in Fig. 4(b). There is substantial intraspinal branching of corticospinal axons, which can be visualized by intra-axonal injection of horseradish peroxidase [7]. Much of the branching is within the motor nuclei (Rexed's lamina IX), and is most extensive in the rostro-caudal direction, i.e. in parallel with the columns of motoneurons (Fig. 4b).

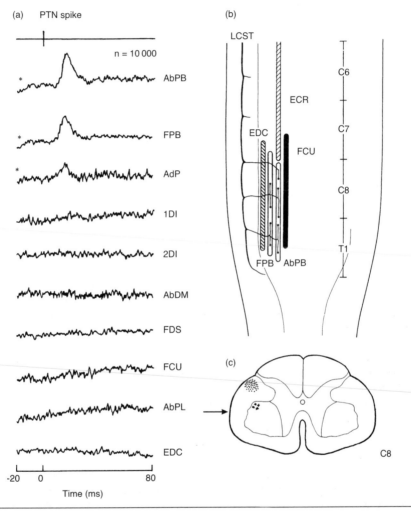

Fig. 4. (a) Distribution of post-spike facilitation from single CM cells to muscles of the hand and forearm in the monkey and (b) schematic horizontal section, at the level indicated by the arrow in (c), through the monkey lower cervical cord showing a relatively restricted output from the axon of a single CM cell running in the lateral corticospinal tract (LCST), and with collaterals contacting motoneuron cell columns innervating two thumb muscles (FPB and AbPB), but not a finger extensor (EDC), wrist extensor (ECR) or flexor (FCU)

(a) Spike-triggered averages of EMG activity recorded concurrently from 10 muscles and averaged with respect to 10000 spikes from a PTN, which discharged at time zero. All data were recorded while the monkey performed the precision grip task. Asterisks indicate averages with clear effects: only three of the muscles (AbPB, FPB and AdP), all acting on the thumb, show definite post-spike facilitation. Reproduced with permission from [4].

For a sample of 80 CM cells active during the precision grip task, the proportion of muscles facilitated by a single cell was found to be fairly restricted: just over a quarter of the muscles sampled yielded PSF. In the example shown in Fig. 4(a), three out of ten muscles were facilitated by the CM cell. PSF in a single intrinsic hand muscle, generally a thumb muscle, was relatively uncommon (19 out of 80 CM cells). It is perhaps to be expected that the thumb should receive the most focused output from the cortex. But given the relatively small number of muscles sampled in these experiments (at most only 10 of the 29 or so acting on the hand and digits) it seems unlikely that a single CM cell controls a single muscle. Control of select groups of muscles is the fundamental organizational principle of the CM projection.

The term 'muscle field' describes the set of muscles innervated by a CM cell [8]. The facilitation by a CM cell of different target muscles is potentially of great functional significance. Since most of the CM cells facilitating hand muscles influence a relatively restricted group of muscles, it seems quite possible that this focused pattern of facilitation contributes to the fractionation of muscle activity necessary for precision finger movements. Indeed, the combination of muscles facilitated by a single CM cell could reflect the anatomical relationship of the target muscles [4]. Thus some cells facilitated both the long extensor of the digits (extensor digitorum communis, EDC) and the intrinsic hand muscle, first dorsal interosseous (1DI). Both muscles are involved in extension of the interphalangeal joints of the index finger, essential during precision grip. Other CM cells had muscle fields which reflected task-related synergies, such as the facilitation of both the 1DI and the thumb adductor, AdP. These muscles are two of the 'prime movers' within the intrinsic group for the production of precision grip.

In another series of studies by Fetz, Cheney and colleagues, it was found that most of the CM cells active during a wrist flexion–extension task, facilitated either wrist flexor or extensor EMG activity [8]. For about a third of these cells, a given neuron facilitated an agonist muscle and suppressed EMG activity in the antagonist muscle. Inhibition must play an important role in the shaping of muscular activity during hand movement.

> ▶ Motor cortex neurons with CM connections have a number of features: (i) they exert powerful facilitation of activity in hand muscles; (ii) they facilitate activity in a small group of muscles (these may be muscles that are functional, but not necessarily anatomical, synergists); (iii) they are particularly active during RIFM; (iv) some cells code for the force exerted during grip; and (v) they receive sensory projections from the hand.

Activity of identified CM cells during skilled hand movements

Monkey CM cells thus have a restricted pattern of connectivity among the spinal motoneuron pools innervating the hand, and this connectivity is well-suited for the recruitment and control of small groups of synergist muscles. Some CM cells facilitating hand muscles are preferentially active in the execution of a precision grip task, requiring fractionation of distal muscle activity and RIFM, as opposed to a power grip in which a co-contracted pattern of muscular activity was needed [4]. The important point here is that the activity of a CM cell, and that of its target muscle, could be dissociated by changing the task performed. Thus despite the direct nature of the CM linkage, the recruitment of CM cells is flexible in nature.

Because of differences in the amplitude of PSF in the different muscles making up the muscle field of a CM cell, it is possible that the CM input could influence the precise balance of fractionated activity across the muscles during RIFM. The selective recruitment of CM cells during finger movement suggests that the pattern of synaptic influence detected by the STA technique can and does contribute to the relative levels of activity in different intrinsic hand muscles during precision grip. The expression of muscle synergies in terms of the synaptic weighting of CM cells may be one means of reducing the large number of possible muscle combinations (or degrees of freedom) with which the motor system has to deal (see above).

The control of force

An important aspect of skilled hand movement is the precise control and co-ordination of force at the finger tips. During skilled prehension tasks, the grip force exerted on an object is carefully adapted to its shape, texture and weight

[9]. There is an accurate co-ordination of the grip force and the load force that must be exerted to lift an object. Many studies have demonstrated the existence of motor cortex neurons whose activity is correlated with force [7]. A particular involvement with fine motor control at low forces is indicated by the finding that many of these neurons are already active at very low force levels, and show rapid changes in firing rate with small increases in force: their activity may saturate at higher force levels, or even decrease. Comparatively few studies have reported neurons that are selectively recruited at high force levels, i.e. in a manner similar to high threshold alpha motoneurons.

When considering the activity in central neural structures that is related to a particular parameter of movement, such as force, direction or velocity, it is important to distinguish activity which may serve as a central representation of the parameters, from that which is causally related to its execution. The former class of activity is probably important for many aspects of voluntary control, including the 'sense of effort' and the construction of an internal representation of limb position and movement [2]. Thus neuronal activity related to force can be demonstrated in several different cortical areas, but not all of this activity will be directly concerned with commands to motoneurons and muscles to provide the appropriate level of contraction. For this type of activity it is of particular importance to know something about the parametric relations of identified output neurons, including CM cells.

The discharge rate of CM cells facilitating wrist muscles shows a monotonic relationship with force exerted at the wrist [8]. However, quite different results were found for CM cells facilitating intrinsic hand muscles, and whose firing rate was investigated in relation to level of static force exerted by monkeys performing the precision grip task [7]. Surprisingly, only one-third of the CM cells analysed showed significant positive correlations with grip force. The activity of some cells had a significant negative correlation with force, despite the fact that these cells clearly had an excitatory influence over their target muscles. These negatively co-varying motor cortex cells have not been found in studies of force control involving other tasks, such as jaw, wrist or forearm movements [7]. The decreasing activity of such cells at higher forces could reflect a reduced drive to spinal

mechanisms that usually promote reciprocal inhibition of antagonist muscles, thus allowing the co-contraction required for precision grip to occur. Alternatively the activity of these cells could reflect peripheral feedback from the gripping skin surfaces at the fingertips. Finally, such cells could provide a sensitive mechanism for the controlled release of objects from the grip, since they would be most active at very low force levels, when the discharge rate of neurons whose activity positively co-varies with force would be declining.

Correlations with static precision grip force were more common for CM cells with slowly conducting axons than with rapidly conducting axons. One could speculate and suggest that the CM cells with fast-conducting axons (the classical 'fast' pyramidal tract neurons, PTNs) are particularly important for 'shaping' the pattern of muscle activity during RIFM, while the 'slow' PTNs may contribute to the background drive to the motoneuron pool, essential for control of hand posture and grip force. In the human pyramidal tract, PTNs with small, slowly conducting axons probably outnumber the large, faster ones by a factor of ten to one [7].

Electrophysiological measurements suggest that a number of CM cells converge upon a single alpha motoneuron. These cells are referred to collectively as the CM 'colony' for that motoneuron. Presumably a substantial proportion of the colony must be activated simultaneously to provide a significant CM drive to the motoneuron.

The importance of sensory feedback to the motor cortex

Sensory feedback is of obvious importance for skilled motor control. When lifting small objects, subtle changes in object texture lead to a readjustment of the grip force to prevent it slipping from the grip, but this effect disappears when the fingertips are anaesthetized [9]. A number of studies of patients with a complete peripheral neuropathy have shown that while simple motor acts (the generation of constant force or position with the hand, for instance) can be carried out by such patients without any feedback, all complex acts involving the hand were severely affected, and could only be performed with the assistance of vision after lengthy retraining [10]. Interestingly, monkeys with pyramidal tract section show problems of tactile placing and these deficits in digit control resemble those observed after section of the dorsal column sensory pathways. These observations stress the importance of sensory-motor integration for normal manipulative skills.

The majority of motor cortex neurons receive feedback from the periphery, and this includes output elements such as PTNs and CM cells. While much of this feedback appears to come from muscle receptors, for those neurons active during hand and finger movements a substantial proportion receive their input from specific afferent input zones on the glabrous skin of the hand. The activity of these neurons can vary with the texture of the gripped object.

The pathways mediating these peripheral inputs to the motor cortex are still not fully understood. There are fast pathways that gain access to area 4 directly from the thalamus, and others that relay through areas 3a, 2 and 5. The 3a projection is probably most important for the input from muscle receptors. In the primate, there are few direct projections from areas 3b and 1, and the major projection appears to come from the 'higher order' areas 2 and 5, where neurons with complex sensory receptive fields are found. Interestingly, patients with posterior parietal lesions have striking deficits of skilled finger movement [11].

Organization of the motor cortex outputs to the hand

How are cortical outputs represented in the 'motor map' at the cortical level? Detailed investigation of the fine structure of this map have demonstrated that rather than consisting of a simple somatotopic representation of muscles, the map contains the building blocks of complex movements, i.e. those requiring activation of multiple muscles. First, there is a multiple representation of a given muscle over an extensive region of the primary motor cortex. This representation is often discontinuous. Multiple representation may well reflect the many different combinations in which a muscle can be used during a voluntary movement. Since the muscles of the hand have the most varied uses, it is not surprising to find that their representation is the most extensive. Secondly, there is a very substantial overlap between the outputs directed to different muscles. To some extent, this is provided for by the divergent axons of individual CM cells, as described earlier. But there are, in addition, clusters of cortical output neurons with quite different muscle fields. These clusters, which are available for selection by input systems to the motor cortex, appear to be the cortical representation of the functional muscular synergies that underly skilled movement.

▶ The organization of the motor cortex involves input and output maps.
▶ The input map represents the spatial and type of sensory input from the periphery.
▶ The output map represents the muscles and movements.
▶ The selection of outputs by different inputs generates a functional map.

In addition to the large hand and digit regions within the output map, there are significant representations of muscles acting at more proximal joints: shoulder, elbow and wrist. But the overlapping nature of these outputs suggests that they act together to produce a suitable posture and direction of arm movement that is essential for the successful execution of a skilled hand movement. Observation of a skilled pianist or violinist provides a striking example of this point.

Recent work shows the output map of the motor cortex to be a dynamic one. It may undergo significant change when the target motoneurons are disrupted, or afferent inputs disturbed, for instance after congenital amputation [7,12]. Further striking changes have been demonstrated after stroke affecting the major output pathways from the motor cortex [13]. These changes reveal an important capacity for reorganization that may assist in the recovery that so often follows brain damage. The results represent an exciting challenge for those interested in applying the important knowledge gained from animal experiments to the assessment and therapy of brain-damaged patients with motor disorders.

▶ The output map has a number of important features: (i) there is multiple representation of a given muscle; (ii) there is extensive overlap between the representation of different muscles; and (iii) the map is a dynamic map, it can show some degree of reorganization as the result of motor learning or in response to injury.

References

1. Rosenbaum, D.A. (1991) Human Motor Control, Academic Press, New York
2. Kalaska, J.F. and Crammond, D.J. (1992) Cerebral cortical mechanisms of reaching movements. Science **255**, 1517–1523
3. Dum, R.P. and Strick, P.L. (1991) The origin of corticospinal projections from the premotor areas in the frontal lobe. J. Neurosci. **11**, 667–689
4. Lemon, R.N. (1993) Cortical control of the primate hand. The 1992 G.L. Brown Prize Lecture. Exp. Physiol. **78**, 263–301
5. Rothwell, J.C., Thompson, P.D., Day, B.L., Boyd, S. and Marsden, C.D. (1991) Stimulation of the human motor cortex through the scalp. Exp. Physiol. **76**, 159–200
6. Armand, J. (1982) The origin, course and terminations of corticospinal fibers in various mammals. Prog. Brain Res. **57**, 330–360
7. Porter, R. and Lemon, R.N. (1993) Corticospinal Function and Voluntary Movement, Oxford University Press, Oxford
8. Cheney, P.D., Fetz, E.E. and Mewes, K. (1991) Neural mechanisms underlying corticospinal and rubrospinal control of limb movements. Prog. Brain Res. **87**, 213–252
9. Johansson, R.S. (1991) How is grasping modified by somatosensory input? In: Motor Control: Concepts and Issues (Humphrey, D.R. and Freund, H.-J., eds.), pp. 331–356, Wiley, Chichester
10. Rothwell, J.C., Traub, M.M., Day, B.L., Obeso, J.A., Thomas, P.K. and Marsden, C.D. (1982) Manual motor performance in a deafferented man. Brain **105**, 515–542
11. Pause, M., Kunesch, E., Binkofski, F. and Freund, H.-J. (1989) Sensorimotor disturbances in patients with lesions of the parietal cortex. Brain **112**, 1599–1625
12. Pons, T.P., Garraghty, P.E., Ommaya, A.K., Kaas, J.H., Taub, E. and Mishkin, M. (1991) Massive cortical reorganization after sensory deafferentation in adult macaques. Science **252**, 1857–1860
13. Chollet, F., Dipiero, V., Wise, R.J.S., Brooks, D.J., Dolan, R.J. and Frackowiak, R.S.J. (1991) The functional anatomy of motor recovery after stroke in humans: a study with positron emission tomography. Ann. Neurol. **29**, 265–276

2

The basal ganglia

John C. Rothwell
MRC Human Movement and Balance Unit, Institute of Neurology, Queen Square, London WC1N 3BG, U.K.

Anatomy

The basal ganglia consist of five inter-related nuclei situated in the interior of the cerebral hemispheres and upper midbrain. The main bulk consists of three nuclei, the caudate, putamen and globus pallidus. Phylogenetically, the globus pallidus is the oldest part of the group and is known as the paleostriatum. The caudate and putamen phylogenetically are newer and together are termed the neostriatum (or sometimes just striatum for short). In man, they are divided by the internal capsule. In the rat, they form a single unit. The term striatum is descriptive of their appearance in myelin-stained sections. A number of fibre bundles known as Wilson's pencils traverse the nuclei giving them a striped appearance. The globus pallidus is divided into two parts, the lateral or external part (GPe), and the medial or internal part (GPi), by the medial medullary lamina. The lateral or external part is larger than the medial or internal part. Although both parts look similar, they have connections with quite different parts of the brain.

The remaining two nuclei of the basal ganglia, the substantia nigra and subthalamic nucleus, are smaller but no less important. The substantia nigra is particularly well developed in man and can be seen with the naked eye as a dark stripe above the cerebral peduncle. It is divided into two parts which have separate connections with different parts of the brain. There is no clear demarcation line, but the cells are more densely packed in the dorsal part of the nucleus than in the ventral part, and that area appears darker when examined by eye. The dorsal region is known as the pars compacta (SNpc) and the ventral region as the pars reticulata (SNpr). As we shall see below, the pars reticulata is often regarded as homologous to the GPi, both structures being major output nuclei of the basal ganglia.

The subthalamic nucleus is a small lens-shaped nucleus situated beneath the thalamus. It is a pivotal part of the intrinsic circuitry of the basal ganglia.

Connections of the basal ganglia

The major input to the basal ganglia comes from wide areas of cerebral cortex, and the major output is, via the thalamus, back on to the same areas of cortex. This forms a cortex–basal ganglia–cortex loop. It is only recently that the details of the connections within this pathway have become apparent [1]. They are summarized in Fig. 1. Note that in this Figure, the GPi and SNpr are treated together, even though they are anatomically separate.

The main receiving nuclei of the basal ganglia are the caudate and putamen (striatum); the main output nuclei are the GPi and SNpr. These nuclei send the bulk of their efferent fibres to thalamus and thence to cortex. However, there are several other projection targets which receive a smaller number of fibres including the superior colliculus, reticular formation and the pedunculo-pontine nucleus. The cortical input to the caudate and putamen is excitatory and glutamatergic. Cortical synapses are found on the tips of dendritic spines of medium spiny neurons which comprise more than 90% of the neurons of the striatum [2]. These neurons are both the receiving and projection neurons of the striatum and send axons to the output nuclei (GPi/SNpr) via two separate pathways. Some of the medium spiny neurons project directly to GPi and SNpr. This pathway is GABA-ergic (GABA, γ-amino butyric acid) and inhibitory and co-localizes substance P as a neurotransmitter. The other pathway from striatum to GPi/SNpr is indirect. It takes the route striatum to GPe to subthalamic nucleus to GPi. The projection

from striatum to GPe, like the direct pathway to GPi, is GABA-ergic, but, in this case, enkephalins rather than substance P are co-localized as neurotransmitters. GPe has no direct output to thalamus. Its major projection is to the subthalamic nucleus and thence to GPi/SNpr.

The signs (excitatory or inhibitory) of all the synapses in the basal ganglia pathways are now known and are indicated in Fig. 1. The GABA-ergic pathways are inhibitory whereas the glutamatergic pathways are excitatory. If we follow the inhibitory and excitatory connections of the direct pathway, we find that excitatory cortical input to the striatum produces disinhibition (i.e. two inhibitory

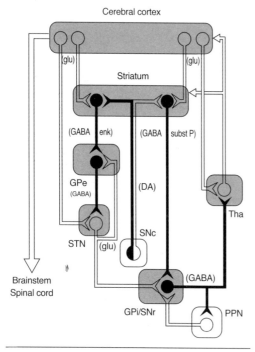

Cerebral cortex

(glu)   (glu)

Striatum

(GABA enk)   (GABA subst P)

GPe
(GABA)

(DA)

Tha

STN   (glu)

SNc

Brainstem
Spinal cord

(GABA)

GPi/SNr   PPN

Fig. I. Schematic diagram of the main circuits and neurotransmitters involved in the cortico-basal ganglia-cortex circuit

Excitatory connections are shown as open neurons, inhibitory connections are shown as filled neurons. Note the 'direct' pathway from striatum to internal globus pallidus (GPi), and the 'indirect' pathway via the external globus pallidus (GPe) and subthalamic nucleus (STN). PPN, pedunculopontine nucleus; SNc, substantia nigra pars compacta (Reproduced with permission from ref. [1]).

synapses) of the thalamus and hence results in excitation back at the cortex. If the synapses in the indirect pathway are followed, it can be seen that information flowing in this route has the opposite effect, and results in an inhibitory effect on the thalamus and cortex. The opposite signs of activity in the direct and indirect pathways through the basal ganglia have led some authors to speculate that they must interact temporally or spatially such that (a) activity in the inhibitory pathway might brake activity in the direct excitatory pathway, or (b) that the inhibitory pathway might produce some form of 'surround inhibition' of activity in the direct pathway.

During its passage through the basal ganglia, input from a wide area of cortex is funnelled through successively smaller structures, and at one time it was thought that inputs from various areas of the brain would converge in some way before the final output was produced. Although such spatial interaction between inputs from different cortical areas is possible anatomically, this does not appear to happen. Under normal circumstances, inputs are kept quite separate through their passage in the basal ganglia, and at present it is believed that the inputs from various cortical regions form separate 'loops' which run in parallel through the basal ganglia circuitry (Fig. 2) [3]. The main loops that concern us here are the motor loop from the sensory-motor cortex (Fig. 2), and the oculomotor loop from frontal areas of cortex involved in eye movements. Even within a major loop, inputs may be kept separate. In the motor loop, inputs from the arm, leg and face intermix very little.

Ideas on the detailed organization of the motor loop are still evolving. Some authors indicate that inputs from all cortical motor areas plus the primary sensory cortex, converge on the same area of striatum. Others (as in Fig. 2) consider only some portions of sensory-motor cortex to be major contributors. In the past, the major output target of the motor loop was believed to be the supplementary motor area. However, this is now considered to be incorrect. Large outputs are also found in the primary motor cortex and the ventral premotor cortex. Indeed, the outputs to supplementary, primary and ventral premotor areas all arise from separate regions of the GPi, suggesting that these may be further functional specializations within the motor loop [4].

▶ The basal ganglia consists of five main subcortical nuclei: caudate, putamen, subthalamic nucleus, substantia nigra and globus pallidus. The latter two are subdivided into two sections each, the substantia nigra pars reticulata (SNpr), substantia nigra pars compacta (SNpc), and the internal and external segments of the globus pallidus (GPi and GPe).

▶ The major flow of information through the basal ganglia is in a cortex–basal ganglia–thalamus–cortex loop. The caudate and putamen receive input from the cortex, and the SNpr and GPi send information back to the thalamus and then to the cortex. In addition, there are some smaller projections to brainstem centres.

▶ There are two parallel information pathways through the basal ganglia: the direct and the indirect route. Information can flow either directly from the receiving nuclei (caudate and putamen) to the output nuclei (GPi and SNpr) or can make a detour via the GPe and subthalamic nucleus.

Dopamine

In addition to their input from cerebral cortex, the neurons of the caudate and putamen receive a dopaminergic input from the SNpc. These dopamine synapses are located at the base of the dendritic spines of medium spiny neurons, and are therefore in a good position to modulate the action of cortical synapses which are found at the tips of each spine [2]. It was once unclear whether dopamine had an excitatory or inhibitory action on striatal neurons. The answer now appears to be both. It has opposite actions on the neurons of the direct and indirect pathways (see Fig. 1). Dopaminergic input is inhibitory on neurons of the indirect pathway which project from striatum to GPe (perhaps via the D2 receptor type), and excitatory on neurons which project directly to GPi/SNpr (perhaps via a D1 receptor subtype).

The dopaminergic cells of the SNpc receive input from the caudate and putamen. However, this input is separate from the main flow of information from striatum to GPi/SNpr. It is discussed in the next section.

Striosomes

In addition to the parallel loop organization of the basal ganglia, there is, in the striatum, another less well understood form of organization [5]. Despite their homogenous appearance, the medium spiny neurons of the caudate and putamen appear to form two distinct sub-populations. These sub-populations do not correspond to neurons which form the direct and indirect output pathways. They have been identified with various techniques, and have been given different names according to which technique was used to separate them. Thus, some authors have described 'islands' of more densely packed cells within a matrix of less dense packing. Other authors have seen groups of cells ('striosomes') which stain less densely for acetylcholinesterase than the cells which surround them. Finally, some groups have described 'patches' of neurons rich in opiate receptors. It is thought that all three techniques identify the same clusters of neurons, and it has been proposed that these clusters should be known as striosomes. The remainder of the cells in the striatum are termed the matrix.

In the motor loop through the basal ganglia, the main striatal target of sensory-motor input is matrix (mostly putamen). Input to the striosomal compartment comes mostly from limbic structures. Interestingly, there is a striatal projection to dopaminergic cells of the SNpc. This also arises from the striosomal component rather than the matrix, even though both receive dopaminergic input. Thus, it is the limbic areas of cortex which, by their input to the striosomes, have direct access to the dopaminergic cells of the SNpc. Since these dopaminergic cells project back to the matrix, the implication is that emotional/attentional factors may influence transmission through the basal ganglia motor loop [2].

▶ The caudate and putamen are not homogenous structures. They can be divided, on the basis of the density of certain neurotransmitters into striosomes and matrix.

▶ The major receiving areas for sensory-motor input are matrix. The striosomal compartment receives input from many other areas including the limbic system.

▶ Some of the striosomal output projects to the dopaminergic cells of the SNpc which in turn project back on to the neurons of the matrix compartment. This is a possible route whereby emotional factors may influence performance in the motor parts of the basal ganglia.

Electrophysiology

There are two features of basal ganglia discharge which have had an important influence on theories of basal ganglia function. First, the major output from the GPi and SNpr to thalamus is inhibitory. Secondly, at rest, these cells fire at sustained high frequencies [6]. In contrast, there is very little, if any, spontaneous dis-

charge in the cells of the caudate and putamen. Such continuous tonic inhibitory output of the basal ganglia at rest has given rise to the idea that removal of this inhibition might somehow 'allow' movement to occur. However, precisely what aspect of movement might be 'allowed' is very much debated. Recordings of the activity of single neurons during different types of movement in monkeys have given rise to several theories of the possible role of the basal ganglia.

Many neurons in the basal ganglia change their firing pattern in relation to active movements of the contralateral side of the body. Unlike, for example, neurons in the primary motor cortex, the firing of neurons in the basal ganglia (mostly recorded in the putamen or globus pallidus) (a) occurs late relative to the onset of movement, and (b) is related best to the direction of movement rather than the pattern

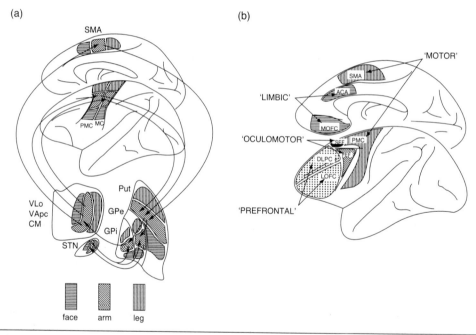

(a)   (b)

Fig. 2. (a) Diagram of the motor loop through the basal ganglia, showing that the somatotopic subdivisions of the input remain separate throughout the circuit and (b) areas of the frontal lobes which receive output from separate basal ganglia circuits

(b) Targets of four different basal ganglia-cortex 'loops' are shown: the motor loop (MC, primary motor cortex; PMC, premotor cortex; SMA, supplementary motor area), the oculomotor loop (SEF, supplementary eye fields; FEF, frontal eye fields), the limbic loop (ACA, ante-rior cingulate area; MOFC, medial orbitofrontal cortex), and the frontal loop (DLPC, dorsolateral prefrontal cortex; LOFC, lateral orbitofrontal cortex) (Reproduced with permission from ref. [1]).

of muscle activity necessary to achieve it [6]. Thus, in a reaction time task, in which a monkey makes a limb movement after some sensory 'go' signal, the majority of globus pallidus or putamenal cells change their discharge rate after movement has begun. This compares with the 50% or so of cells in the primary motor cortex which discharge prior to the onset of movement. The late discharge of basal ganglia neurons may therefore reflect the fact that their major input comes from sensorimotor areas of cortex. The relationship of the firing pattern to the direction of limb movement is illustrated in Fig. 3. In this experiment, a monkey made elbow flexion movements against either an opposing or an assisting load. In such tasks, the pattern of electromyographic (EMG) activity can be dissociated from the direction of movement. With an opposing load, the movement is made using agonist activity, whereas with an assisting load, the movement is made using the braking action of the antagonist. In the putamen, a minority of the neurons have a discharge which reflects the pattern of EMG activity, while most of them discharge according to the direction of movement. This is also true for globus pallidus and subthalamic neurons.

The implication of these results is that the basal ganglia discharge is unlikely to be intimately involved in either the onset of a movement, or in specifying the precise pattern of muscle activity needed to achieve it. Several authors have taken these facts and added further observations of their own in order to develop hypotheses of the possible role of the basal ganglia in control of movement.

Hypothesis I
The basal ganglia work by disinhibiting areas of the motor system and thus 'allow' movement to

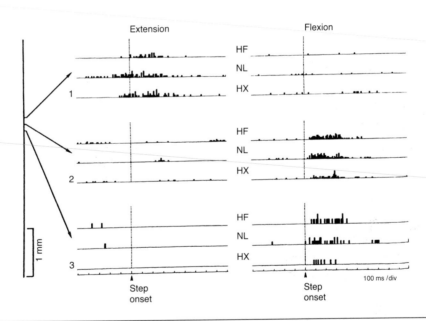

Fig. 3. Relationship between firing frequency and direction of elbow movement in three different neurons encountered during the course of a single microelectrode penetration (left) through the monkey putamen

The task was to flex (right) or extend (left) the elbow rapidly in response to movement of a visual target. Movements were made either with no load (NL), with a constant load (150 g) opposing flexion (HF), or with a load opposing extension (HX). Histograms of average unit activity for each cell in the six different tasks are shown. Vertical broken line indicates time of onset of movement. The first neuron (1) was active during extension movements, whereas the other two neurons (2 and 3) were active during flexion movements. Thus, activity was related to direction in these cells, but not the force of movement. (Reproduced with permission from ref. [7]).

occur. In this hypothesis [8], removal of tonic basal ganglia inhibition may facilitate movements, but may not be absolutely necessary for movement to occur. Movement may still be made in the absence of changes in the basal ganglia activity, although with more 'difficulty' than usual.

Much of the work to support this hypothesis comes from the study of eye movements [9], and hence involves the oculomotor loop through the basal ganglia. Many areas of the cerebral cortex are involved in control of eye movements (for example, the frontal eye fields, supplementary eye fields, dorsolateral prefrontal cortex and the posterior parietal cortex). Cells in these areas project to the caudate nucleus whence they influence activity in the SNpr and GPi. Their output is back to the cortex via the thalamus, and also, from the SNpr to the superior colliculus, an area in the brainstem intimately involved in the production of eye movements.

Fig. 4 shows the pattern of neural firing during a visually guided saccadic eye movement made by a monkey. The monkey fixated a visual target which then jumped to the left or the right. After a reaction time of about 200 ms, the eyes move rapidly to recapture the target on the fovea. The discharge of cells in the SNpr is relatively high prior to target movement, but some 100 ms or so after the target moves, their discharge decreases dramatically. Shortly after this, the neurons of the superior colliculus, which usually have a low tonic firing rate, suddenly increase their discharge. Examining the circuitry of the basal ganglia, we can see that the results can be explained by postulating that the tonic output of the SNpr is inhibitory to the superior colliculus, and that its removal 'allows' the collicular cells to fire.

Such an effect of nigral disinhibition on superior colliculus cell firing can be observed pharmacologically. Injection of the excitatory neurotransmitter glutamate into the striatum of a rat can cause an increase in firing of striatal cells. This results, by way of the inhibitory projection to the SNpr, in a decrease in the tonic firing rate of the SNpr cell. At the same time there is an increase in the firing rate of cells in the superior colliculus (and thalamus).

In the example shown in Fig. 4, the burst of collicular firing is necessary to produce saccadic eye movements; movement will not occur if the superior collicular cells do not discharge. The

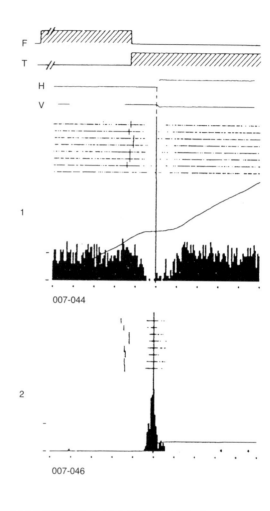

007-044

007-046

Fig. 4. Activities of a neuron in the substantia nigra pars reticulata (1), and one of its presumed target cells in the superior colliculus (2) during a visually guided saccadic eye movement in a monkey

The traces in the upper part of the Figure illustrate the target and eye movements. The top trace shows the duration of the fixation point display (F), the second trace the time of appearance of the target (T), and the third trace shows when the horizontal eye movement began (H). The trace labelled V shows the vertical component of the eye movement. The accompanying neuronal discharges in the nigra and colliculus are shown both as dot raster displays and time histograms. The nigral cell discharges at a high rate during fixation, but is suppressed just before the onset of the saccade. At the same time, the collicular cell fires. After completion of the saccade, the basal firing rates in each structure are resumed. (Reproduced with permission from ref. [9]).

situation is different for the changes observed in SNpr discharge. Eye movements are not an obligatory consequence of a decrease in nigral cell firing. There are occasions when eye movements occur without any observable change in basal ganglia firing; conversely changes in nigral discharge can be observed without any concommitant eye movement.

An example of this type of behaviour occurs when monkeys make saccades to 'remembered' targets. In these experiments, the animal is trained to fixate a central spot while a target is presented briefly in the periphery. However, the monkey has not to move his eyes to the target until the central fixation spot is blanked out. At this time, the target has disappeared, hence the description that the saccades were made to a 'remembered' target. Under these conditions, some nigral cells decrease their discharge rate soon after target presentation and retain that low firing rate until the saccade is made. It is as though the SNpr were facilitating or 'preparing' the colliculus until such time as the saccade was released.

Hypothesis 2

The basal ganglia are involved in turning off 'automatic' postural activity so that voluntary movement can occur. They also prevent the appearance of unwanted movements during focal tasks. This is the hypothesis of Mink and Thach [10]. It differs from the hypothesis outlined above in two respects: (1) it proposes a more important role for the basal ganglia in the control of postural muscle activity than in producing activity in the prime mover, and (2) it emphasizes the prevention of movement, and as such, it implies that the important change in basal ganglia output during movement is an increase, and not a decrease, in pallidal discharge.

Mink and Thach [10] examined the discharge of pallidal neurons during many different types of movement: fast, slow, visually guided and self-paced, and they concluded that the neuronal discharge was unrelated to any particular parameters of movement. Even though the discharge, as reported by others, was directionally selective in some tasks, this was not a consistent finding. They found that directional preference could vary in different tasks.

Because of the variability in the neuronal discharge, these authors did not attempt to correlate different patterns of neural firing with different types of movement. Instead, they used another approach. They inactivated pallidal neurons by injecting small amounts of kainic acid in order to inactivate cells without disrupting activity in fibres of passage. Thus, the authors could observe the effects of lack of pallidal discharge on movement control. They found that the effect was very similar to that seen in basal ganglia diseases in man. (1) When movements were made there was inappropriate co-contraction of antagonist muscles; (2) the monkeys tended to assume a flexed posture; (3) their movements were slow; and (4) the animals had difficulties in turning off muscle activity (e.g. in movements made with an assisting load where antagonist activity has to be turned off before movement can begin).

The interpretation is that the basal ganglia are not intimately involved in control of the prime moving muscle, but primarily influence the 'automatic' postural activity in other muscles. Failure to switch off the activity leads to co-contraction and a flexed posture. Without the appropriate braking action of the basal ganglia, movements are not easily released, and tend to be slow. It must be stressed that this hypothesis, unlike hypothesis 1, involves increased basal ganglia output during movement, and that this is used to switch off unwanted muscle activity.

Hypothesis 3

Alexander and Crutcher [3] have suggested that it may be inappropriate to imagine that the basal ganglia only perform one specific function. The very range of cell firing behaviour which is observed may reflect the fact that a range of different processes are being performed simultaneously. In their experiments, they used opposing or assisting loads to dissociate direction-related from muscle-related activity. In addition, they could dissociate the direction of target movement from the direction of limb movement, so that, for example, in order to move the target from the right to the left, the monkey had to flex his wrist to the right. Finally, they examined cell firing in (i) the preparatory period before a movement when monkeys might have been given information on, say, the direction of the upcoming movement, but not told exactly when it was to occur, and (ii) during the execution phase of movement. A large range of neuronal firing patterns occurred. However, there was a tendency for the cell discharges to fall into two groups: those cells which discharged in the preparatory period, after presentation of the instruction stimulus, and those which discharged during execution of the movement itself. In general, the cells which changed their firing pattern in the preparatory period were more likely to be related to the direction of the forthcoming movement or even the direction of the target movement than to the muscle force needed to make the movement. In contrast, cells which changed firing in the execution phase were more likely to be related to movement direction or muscle force.

Alexander and Crutcher [3] also examined neuronal discharge in two cortical motor areas in the same tasks. The range of activity in the supplementary and primary motor areas was essentially similar to that described in the pallidum, although the primary motor cortex tended to have a larger proportion of movement-related cells than preparatory cells, while the opposite was true for the supplementary motor area.

In reviewing their data, Alexander and Crutcher [3] suggested (1) that the sub-populations of cells related to preparatory and execution phases of movement might form two separate sub-channels through the motor loop. Information related to movement preparation may therefore be treated separately from that related to movement performance. In particular, since many cells in primary motor cortex are related to execution of a movement while in supplementary motor cortex there are more preparatory cells, one possibility is that these channels may correspond to the separate pallidal outputs to primary and non-primary motor areas described recently by Hoover and Strick [4]. (2) Within these two sub-populations, groups of cells may have quite different relationships to the parameters of movement, firing according to the direction of target movement, intended movement or muscle activity. These cells are all firing at the same time and similar groups of cells can be found in both basal ganglia and cortical motor areas. Alexander and Crutcher compared the activity with that seen in a parallel computer. Their idea is that the brain may not work in a serial fashion. In other words, it does not (1) identify the position of the target then (2) work out in which direction

to move in order to achieve it, and finally (3) decide what level of muscle activity is needed to move the limbs. Instead, the brain may be performing all three functions at once.

Hypothesis 4

The basal ganglia are involved in execution of sequences of movements. They play a role in (1) performance of 'most automatic' movements, and (2) in changes from one subunit of a sequence to the next.

Brotchie et al. [11] again began with the observation that there is no clear relationship between basal ganglia discharge and parameters of movement. Because of this they developed a more complex task in which monkeys had to perform a sequence of wrist movements consisting of jumps either to the right or left (or vice versa) each separated by a short holding phase.

They emphasized two findings in their experiments. The first was that pallidal discharges were usually most prominent in trials in which movements were predictable and which were performed by the monkeys with the least error. For example, when monkeys began a new block of trials, the discharge in the pallidum might be only weakly modulated, but would increase on subsequent repetitions of the movement. The authors hypothesized that basal ganglia activity was greatest during movements made with the least conscious intervention. Tasks which were difficult or unpredictable (such as those which the monkey had not performed before) would require more conscious intervention and it was these which had the smallest changes in basal ganglia activity. Thus, their first idea was that as movements become more and more 'automatic', control is passed from a conscious, presumably cortical level, to basal ganglia structures.

The second finding that they emphasized was that in a sequence of two movements, some cells had a small burst of firing just before the onset of the second movement. This burst was related both to the timing of the movement and also, in some cases, to its direction. If the monkey could not predict the time or direction of the second movement this burst did not occur. In the authors' terms, it may have been an internal signal indicating a transition between subunits in the sequence.

▶ The neurons of the basal ganglia output nuclei (SNpr and GPi) have a high baseline firing rate and are inhibitory to their target neurons in the thalamus. Since the thalamic output to sensorimotor areas of cortex is excitatory, basal ganglia output is thought to have a tonic (braking) action on the motor system. Manipulation of this tonic inhibitory output may assist the performance of movement in several different ways.

▶ Removal of inhibition may allow movements to occur.

▶ Increasing inhibitory output may stop unwanted movements occurring.

▶ Changing the inhibitory outputs may assist in timing when one movement of a sequence is to stop and the next is to begin.

▶ The output may be more complex than any of the possibilities above and represent the multiple parallel outputs involved in preparation, execution and termination of movement.

Activity in dopaminergic neurons

The dopaminergic neurons of the SNpc have a low resting discharge rate which changes little during different types of movement. However, the cells do show phasic changes in firing rate when novel stimuli are presented during movement, or when food rewards are given. Their discharge does not seem to be related to parameters of movement as such, but to motivational arousal caused by other factors in the environment [12]. As pointed out above, such inputs may provide, via the dopaminergic input into the striatum, a mechanism whereby nonmotor inputs can influence the effectiveness of transmission in the basal ganglia motor loop.

N-Methyl-4-phenyl-1,2,3,6-tetra-hydropyridine (MPTP)

MPTP was first discovered when a group of young drug abusers on the west coast of the United States of America suddenly developed severe Parkinsonian symptoms following self-administration of a batch of synthetic narcotics. It was later discovered that the batch was contaminated with MPTP and that when this sub-stance was given to primates it caused a profound Parkinsonian state similar to that of human Parkinson's disease. MPTP was later found to be a specific toxin which destroyed the dopaminergic cells of the SNpc with remarkably high specificity. Although high doses also affect dopaminergic and noradrenergic neurons in other areas, the effect of low doses is almost completely limited to the SNpc.

Such specific destruction of the dopaminergic innervation of the striatum in an animal model has proved useful in determining the possible role of dopamine in the basal ganglia circuitry. Two changes in basal ganglia discharge have been noted after administration of MPTP to monkeys [13]. (1) The resting discharge of cells in the GPi is increased, and (2) cells are less selective than normal in their response to peripheral input. In normal animals, many basal ganglia cells receive somatosensory input, mostly from deep receptors activated by passive movement of joints on the contralateral side of the body. After administration of MPTP, the receptive field of these neurons is increased dramatically, and the cells may even respond to inputs from both sides of the body. It is thought that dopamine may play a role in maintaining the parallel loop organization of the basal ganglia.

Models of basal ganglia disease in man

Human basal ganglia disease is characterized either by an excess of involuntary movement (hyperkinesias, such as is seen in chorea and ballism) or by a lack of spontaneous or associated movements (hypokinesia, such as seen in patients with Parkinson's disease). As emphasized above, some authors consider that the inhibitory output of the basal ganglia must be removed for movement to occur. According to this theory, hyperkinesias are the result of reduced pallidal inhibition. Whereas hypokinesia is caused by overactive pallidal inhibition. Other authors suggest the opposite, that in order for voluntary movement to be released, automatic postural contractions must be turned off by increased pallidal output. This predicts that hyperkinesias should occur because of overactive pallidal inhibition whereas hypokinesias result from reduced pallidal output.

At the present time there is no special reason to favour one hypothesis over the other. Indeed, it seems most likely that the truth may be a combination of the two, i.e. that the prime movement may be facilitated by decreased pallidal inhibition while at the same time, postural and other activity may be reduced by increased output from other regions of the pallidum. Nevertheless, many proponents of the first hypothesis have stressed the simplicity of their theory by pointing out how easily it may account for many types of hyper- and hypokinesias in basal ganglia disease. The arguments are given below.

(1) Ballism occurs after lesions of the subthalamic nucleus and is characterized by uncontrollable, rapid movements of the contralateral arm and (less frequently) leg. In the model of Fig. 1, we see that removal of the subthalamic nucleus will result in a loss of excitatory input to the internal pallidal segment and the substantia pars reticulata. Effectively this will reduce the inhibitory output of the basal ganglia, and perhaps therefore release extra, unwanted movement.

(2) Chorea is a major symptom of Huntington's disease. The excessive, involuntary movements are usually said to be less abrupt and wild than those of ballism, but this is not always the case. In the early stages of Huntington's disease, when chorea is most prominent, post-mortem brain studies have shown a selective loss in the GABA/enkephalin projection from the striatum to the external pallidal segment. In the model of Fig. 1 this will result in less inhibition of the external pallidal cells and hence to increased inhibition of the subthalamic nucleus. If we imagine excessive inhibition of the subthalamic nucleus to produce an effect similar to a lesion of the same structure, then it is easy to see how excessive movement may occur. The model also helps explain why injection of bicuculline, a GABA-receptor antagonist, into the external pallidal segment can produce chorea in the monkey. The injection blocks striatal inhibition of neurons in the external pallidum. These neurons will therefore increase their firing and produce inhibition of the subthalamic nucleus as proposed for Huntington's disease.

(3) In Parkinson's disease, there is selective degeneration of the dopaminergic innervation of the striatum from the SNpc. In the model, we can see that this should have two effects: removal of dopaminergic excitation of the projection to the GPi and removal of dopaminergic inhibition of the projection to the GPe. Since the striato-pallidal pathway is inhibitory to both external and internal segments, this leads to excessive inhibition of the external pallidum and a reduction of inhibition of the internal pallidum. Following the indirect pathway further, the decreased external pallidal activity results in over-activity in the subthalamic nucleus and hence excessive facilitation of the GPi. Thus the internal pallidum is over-active because of reduced inhibition through the direct route and extra facilitation to the indirect route. Such extra inhibitory output from the basal ganglia may prevent spontaneous and associated movement leading to hypokinesia.

As noted above MPTP poisoning has the same consequence as Parkinson's disease in man. In this case, it has been possible to verify electrophysiologically that such changes in neuronal firing in the external and internal pallidum actually do occur as predicted by the model. In addition, the postulated role of the subthalamic nucleus in contributing to the extra activity of the internal pallidum has led to the discovery that lesions of the subthalamic nucleus in MPTP-induced parkinsonism can alleviate most of the symptoms of that condition (Fig. 5). Such a discovery is important because of the possibility of developing new surgical or pharmacological treatments of Parkinson's disease which involve inactivation of the subthalamic nucleus [14].

Although the model is remarkably effective in some respects, it should always be clear that it is only a model and as such cannot explain everything. For example, pallidal lesions alone never give rise to involuntary movement as they should if the model were completely correct. Indeed, large pallidal lesions in animals produce hypokinesia and are therefore more readily explained by the second hypothesis [12] described above. Despite this, pallidal lesions of the past have been used as a treatment for Parkinson's disease. The balance between hypo- and hyper-kinesia may therefore not be as simple as the model may lead us to believe.

▶ Basal ganglia diseases are accompanied by either an excess (hyperkinesia) or a reduction (hypokinesia) in the number of spontaneous movements.

▶ One model of basal ganglia function postulates that hypokinesia results from an excess of basal ganglia output whereas hyperkinesia results from a reduction in basal ganglia output.

▶ Increased basal ganglia output can be obtained by lesioning the subthalamic nucleus, and such a procedure has been shown to be effective in reversing the hypokinesia seen in experimental animals rendered parkinsonian by administration of the toxin MPTP.

Parkinson's disease

Parkinson's disease is the commonest disease of the basal ganglia. Histologically, there is degeneration of dopaminergic neurons in the SNpc and a concomitant decrease in the dopaminergic innervation of the striatum. Interestingly, for symptoms to appear, more than 80% of the dopaminergic neurons must degenerate. If more than 20% are intact, then it seems that the nervous system can compensate for the deficiency. Degeneration is seen in parts of the brain other than the SNpc, but this is not substantial and it is believed that the major symptoms of the condition are due to dopaminergic deficiencies. This is supported by the success of l-dopa replacement therapy in its treatment.

The physiology of movement control in Parkinson's disease has been investigated in great detail. However, of the classic triad of clinical symptoms (akinesia/bradykinesia, rigidity and tremor), only akinesia/bradykinesia is well explained by current concepts of basal ganglia function.

The terms akinesia/bradykinesia refer to several related deficits of movement in Parkinson's disease. These are: (1) a lack of spontaneous movement, especially noticeable as an immobile and mask-like expression of the face; (2) a lack of associated movements (such as swinging the arms when walking); (3) an increase in reaction time to external stimuli; (4) slowness of movements; (5) a tendency to make smaller movements than required (for instance, small steps when walking or small movements of the pen when writing — micrographia); (6) fatiguability of repetitive movements, as seen, for example, in tapping the hands for any length

of time; and (7) difficulty in performing two different movements at the same time (for instance, rising from a chair to shake hands is performed by normal individuals in one continuous action, whereas a patient with Parkinson's disease will first rise from his chair and only then will he extend his hand in greeting).

Strictly speaking, akinesia should be defined as lack of spontaneous or associated movement. Bradykinesia refers to the slowness of voluntary movement. Most studies have examined deficits in reaction time and movement times during different voluntary tasks performed by the upper limb.

Reaction time

Reaction time can be measured under many different conditions, but in general, the deficits which are seen in Parkinson's disease are relatively small, especially when compared with the changes which occur in the speed of voluntary movement. This is consistent with electrophysiological studies in animals which show that basal ganglia activity generally appears after onset of movement, and hence cannot be of great importance in timing the onset of voluntary movement.

Most studies to date have concluded that compared with normal subjects, the simple reaction time in patients with Parkinson's disease is increased while the choice reaction time is much less affected. In the former task, subjects know in advance which movement to make, and then execute it when a 'go' signal is given. In the latter task, they do not know in advance which one (of two or more) movements may be required. The 'go' signal indicates both the time at which the movement must begin as well as which movement must be performed. For example, in a two choice task, a red light may indicate move to the right, while a green light may indicate move to the left.

In normal subjects, the choice reaction time is much longer than simple reaction time because in the latter condition, subjects can prepare some aspects of the movement in advance. This is thought to decrease the preparatory time for movement and hence to decrease reaction time. The deficit seen in the simple reaction time of patients with Parkinson's disease is usually interpreted as a deficiency in making use of advance information so that the simple reaction time is often not much different to the choice reaction time. In terms of the electrophysio-

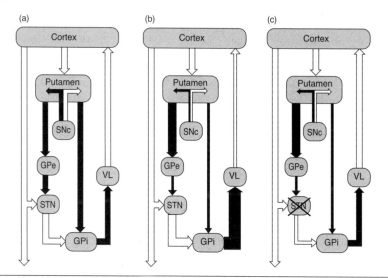

Fig. 5. (a) Normal connectivity in the cortico-basal ganglia-cortex circuit and (b) the situation in MPTP-induced parkinsonism; (c) shows how this situation can be normalized by lesioning the subthalamic nucleus

(a) Open arrows are excitatory connections, filled arrows are inhibitory connections. Note the direct pathway from putamen to internal globus pallidus (GPi) and the indirect pathway via the external pallidus (GPe) and subthalamic nucleus (STN). VL, ventrolateral nuclear region of the thalamus. (b) Degeneration of the dopaminergic projection from the substantia nigra pars compacta (SNc) leads to underactivity in the indirect pathway (thin arrow from striatum to GPi), and overactivity in the output of the indirect pathway from STN to GPi (thick open arrow). The result is excessive activity in the output neurons of the GPi (thick filled arrow), and a reduction in the final excitatory output from thalamus to cortex. (c) Less excitatory drive in the indirect pathway to GPi leads to a reduction in the pallidal inhibition of ventrolateral thalamus. (Reproduced with permisssion from ref. [14]).

logical results discussed above, this might be understood on the basis that changes in basal ganglia output may facilitate motor structures making them more readily activated by other inputs. Perhaps with advance information, the basal ganglia discharge changes before movement, and facilitates particular neuronal circuits so that when the 'go' signal is given, the reaction time is reduced. Without this facilitation, simple reaction times are prolonged.

Another line of evidence suggests that preparation for movement is impaired in Parkinson's disease. This comes from studies of the movement-related potential (MRP) which precedes normal self-initiated voluntary movements. The MRP is a slowly rising negative EEG (electroencephalographic) potential which begins up to 1.5 s before a movement. It consists of two main phases: the NS1 (or BP, Bereitschaftspotential) from 1.5 to 0.6 s before movement, and the NS2 which lasts from 0.6 s before movement to movement onset. This activity is recorded from wide areas of scalp but is maximal at the vertex, and is thought to be caused by activity in the supplementary motor area and the motor cortex (bilaterally). The initial portion of the MRP (the NS1 or BP) is smaller in Parkinson's disease than normal. In contrast, the later portion is often larger in patients than in normals. The interpretation of these results is that the initial period of preparation for movement is abnormal in patients, and that this may be due to reduced basal ganglia output to the cortex in the preparatory period. The later increase in the MRP may represent a functional compensation by other circuits such that the movement eventually is made correctly [15].

Movement time

The deficits in movement time in patients with Parkinson's disease can be much more dramatic than those seen in reaction time. For example, in a simple reaction time task involving supination or pronation of the wrist, Evarts et al. [16] found that reaction time increased by an average of 40%, while movement time increased by an average of 184% in patients as compared with a normal group of age-matched subjects.

Fast movements made at a single joint are produced by a very stereotyped pattern of EMG activity in normal subjects. This activity is sometimes known as the ballistic movement or triphasic pattern and consists of a burst of discharge in the agonist muscles followed by a burst in the antagonist and then by a small second burst in the agonist. The agonist burst provides the impulsive force for the movement, and the antagonist burst acts to brake the movement at the intended end point. The function of the second agonist burst is not yet completely clear, although it may be involved in preventing oscillations around the terminal position. The duration of these EMG bursts and their relative latencies are remarkably constant from one individual to another. Because of this, and because the same pattern can be seen even in totally deafferented individuals, the ballistic movement pattern is thought to represent a single central programme of muscle activation.

When patients with Parkinson's disease attempt to make rapid movements at a single joint (such as the elbow or wrist), two striking deficits are seen (see Fig. 6). Their movements are much slower than normal and the size of their movements is smaller. Because of this latter effect, patients often make large amplitude movements in a series of smaller steps. The basic problem appears to be that the amplitude of the first agonist EMG burst is smaller than it should be, and this results in a movement which fails to achieve the final intended end position. Despite this, all other parameters of the EMG activity are quite normal. Thus, it is usually said that the basic mechanism which produces a ballistic movement pattern is quite normal in patients with Parkinson's disease. The deficit occurs in scaling the amplitude of this pattern to match that required in the movement. A similar failure to scale the amplitude of rapid single joint movements is also seen in monkeys when the globus pallidus is inactivated by cooling or by injection of kainic acid [17].

Although deficits in simple movements made about a single joint are easy to measure, it is often found that the impairments on this task are not well correlated with clinical measures of bradykinesia. This is probably because clinical evaluation involves asking patients to perform complex tasks such as touching each finger in turn with the thumb. In fact, when more complex actions are examined quantitatively, additional deficits show up in the performance of parkinsonian patients. These additional deficits often correlate better with clinical measures of bradykinesia than patients' performance in simple movements.

Benecke et al. [18] devised a task which illustrates these phenomena. They asked subjects to sit in a chair with their arm resting on a lightweight manipulandum which allowed free movement at the elbow. At the end of the manipulandum subjects grasped a stiff force transducer between the thumb and the finger. Various combinations of elbow flexion and squeeze were then performed by patients as rapidly as possible in their own time. When patients performed either elbow flexion on its own or squeezing the force transducer on its own, their movements were slower than normal, as expected. However, when they were required to perform both movements together, or first to squeeze the force transducer and then flex the elbow then their performance deteriorated even further. Each individual component of the movement was made even more slowly than usual, and, in the sequential task, there was a much longer interval between the start of the squeeze and the start of the flex than in normal subjects. This extra slowing in complex movements (i.e. performing two movements at the same time or in a rapid sequence) is never seen in normal subjects, and is thought to reflect the clinical problems that the patients have when they try to do more than one thing at once. It indicates that the basal ganglia may have a crucial role to play in the performance of complex movements. Indeed, the increased interval between movements in the sequential task is quite compatible with the role of the basal gan-

(a) Thumb movements

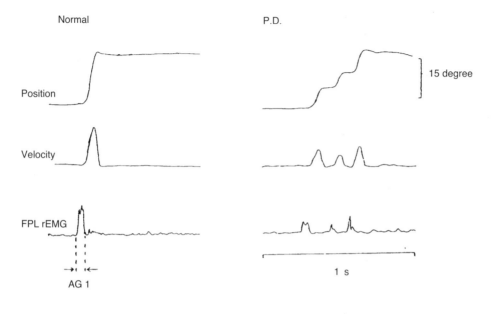

(b) Wrist movements

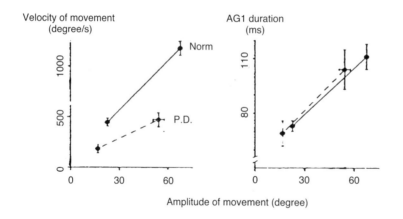

Amplitude of movement (degree)

Fig. 6. Deficits in rapid self-paced thumb (a) and wrist (b) movements in bradykinetic patients with Parkinson's disease

The upper panel shows a representative rapid thumb flexion movement of 20 ° in a normal subject and a patient with Parkinson's disease. The thumb was firmly clamped at the interphalangeal joint so that no postural activity was needed to steady it. The normal subject produces the movement in a single step, using a large burst of EMG activity in the flexor pollicis longus (FPL) muscle. The patient (P.D.) makes the movement in a series of three small steps, with correspondingly small bursts of EMG activity. The bottom panel shows an analysis of similar rapid flexion movements made at the wrist in a group of eight normal and eight patients with Parkinson's disease. Only the initial step of the patients' movements was analysed. The graph on the left shows that movements of a given extent are much slower in patients than normals. However, the duration of the first burst of agonist EMG activity (AG1) was the same (left). This indicates that the basic instructions for the movement were intact. (A. Berardelli, J.C. Rothwell, J.P.R. Dick, B.L. Day and C.D. Marsden, unpublished work).

glia postulated by Brotchie *et al.* [11] in making sequential wrist movements. Perhaps in Parkinson's disease there is a reduction or absence of predictive cell activity signalling the transition between one movement and the next.

A striking feature in Parkinson's disease is the way in which visual input can affect movement. Patients may find it easier to walk along a pattern of stripes painted on the ground than on a plain surface. In contrast, many patients 'freeze' when trying to walk through a doorway. Even if the door is held open, they halt on the threshold and find it impossible to pass through. Their feet appear to be stuck to the ground. Frequently, the only way to get a patient moving again is to use another visual input. Placing one's foot before the patient so that he has to step over it to carry on, usually proves to be effective.

The effect of visual input on movement can be analysed in a laboratory task. Normal subjects and patients with Parkinson's disease can learn to track a moving visual target on a computer screen by moving a joystick backwards or forwards. If a target moves in a predictable way, subjects learn the task and begin to move their joystick in advance of their perception of the target movement. In this way, they can keep up with the target much better than if they were lagging its motion by one reaction time. Parkinsonian subjects are almost as good as normal in learning to predict target motion. However, they fair much worse if the target is blanked from the screen for part of the trial. They may even fail to perform the required movement even though they know what to do. In other words, they are much more dependent on visual feedback to retrieve their movement from memory than normal subjects. In the same way as they fail adequately to use advance information in simple reaction time tasks, during tracking tasks, they have difficulties in accessing stored information about the movement unless visual feedback is allowed.

Tremor and rigidity

Two symptoms of Parkinson's disease are not well understood on current models of basal ganglia function. Unlike spasticity, rigidity is evenly distributed between flexors and extensors. Rigidity describes an increased resistance to passive manipulation of joints. It is caused by a combination of the patient's difficulty in relaxing muscles completely, and also to abnor-

mally enhanced stretch reflex activation of the muscles. There is no evidence for increased excitability of the monosynaptic reflex arc in Parkinson's disease, so that the increased stretch reflex must be due to overactivity in other pathways. Precisely which pathways are involved in producing these increased responses to muscle stretch is not clear. Long-latency stretch reflexes, which can be recorded after sudden, rapid, displacements of a joint are increased in Parkinson's disease. These reflexes, which have an onset latency approximately twice that of the monosynaptic tendon jerk, are produced by activity in a transcortical reflex pathway and also probably by activity in spinal pathways activated by slowly conducting group-II muscle afferents. However, the amount by which the long-latency response is increased does not correlate well in individual patients to the clinically evaluated rigidity. Presumably during clinical testing, which uses rather slow stretches, the reflex response may recruit activity in other, unidentified pathways. How these may be influenced by basal ganglia dysfunction is unknown.

Tremor in Parkinson's disease occurs both at rest and during voluntary activity. Because the frequency of rest tremor (4–6 Hz) is lower than that of action tremor (6–8 Hz) some authors believe them to have different mechanisms [19]. Rest tremor can only be produced in animals by a lesion in the midbrain which damages both the nigro-striatal dopaminergic pathway and the cerebellar outflow pathways to thalamus. Isolated lesions of either group of pathways alone does not result in tremor [20]. The conclusion is that rest tremor in animals does not reflect a pure basal ganglia deficit. The situation is unclear in man. It is usually thought that tremor can occur with isolated damage to the nigro-striatal system. However, there are two pieces of evidence which favour involvement of additional factors. First, it is now possible to measure the activity of the dopaminergic system in man using positron emission tomography (PET) scanning techniques. The degree of deficit in the dopamine system correlates well with clinical measures of rigidity and akinesia, but there is only a very poor correlation, if any, with the amount of tremor. Secondly, it has been known for many years that lesions of the thalamic nucleus Vim (ventralis intermedius) can abolish parkinsonian tremor (and other forms of tremor) very effectively, yet Vim receives no direct basal ganglia input. Although it is possible that the thalamic lesion interrupts fibres of passage from basal ganglia to other thalamic nuclei, it may also indicate a role for other structures in producing the resting tremor of Parkinson's disease.

Postural difficulties

Patients with Parkinson's disease are unstable, especially in the later stages of the disease. A firm, unexpected push to the shoulders may easily overbalance such individuals. Stepping reactions are lost, and there is a failure to throw the limbs out to protect the body during falling. As with tremor and rigidity, it is not clear precisely which deficits in basal ganglia function contribute to these symptoms. One possibility is that control of posture is a function of brainstem structures which project to the spinal cord via the reticulospinal system. If so, then it may be that postural problems result from deficits in the non-thalamic output of basal ganglia. The projection from the GPi and SNpr to the pedunculopontine nucleus, a region in the brainstem known in cats to be involved in locomotion, has been proposed as a possible candidate pathway. Consistent with this, abnormalities in probable reticulospinal function have been recently reported in patients with Parkinson's disease. In rats, and probably in man, the startle response to a sudden unexpected (usually auditory) stimulus arises in the reticular formation and is conducted to the spinal cord in reticulospinal pathways. In patients with Parkinson's disease, the startle response is intact, but the EMG activity occurs slightly later than normal [21]. This has been postulated to result from a lack of tonic influences from the basal ganglia on to brainstem structures. (Note that in this case, the basal ganglia output normally would be expected to facilitate startle mechanisms. If the direct output to brainstem is inhibitory as it is to thalamus and superior colliculus, this would involve another inhibitory connection — i.e. a disinhibition, in order to produce facilitation.)

▶ Parkinson's disease is the commonest disorder of basal ganglia. It results from death of the dopaminergic cells of the substantia nigra pars compacta. These symptoms are caused by lack of dopaminergic innervation to caudate and putamen.

▶ The symptoms are akinesia, tremor, rigidity, and, in the later stages, postural difficulties.

▶ Electrophysiologically, the main abnormality is a slowness of all voluntary movements, particularly if more than one task has to be performed at the same time. In addition, there is an increase in reaction time. Stretch reflexes are increased, and may contribute to the patients' rigidity. Visual input often helps to improve performance.

Chorea

Chorea may result from many different causes, one of the most common of which, and that on which most studies have been performed, is Huntington's disease. This is a dominantly inherited disease with symptoms involving not only chorea but also a progressive decrease in higher cortical function. These symptoms do not appear until about the age of 30–40 years, by which time the next generation usually has been born; 50% of these children will have the disease. At first, involuntary movements and psychiatric changes often begin together. However, chorea gradually becomes more florid until the movements are almost incessant. Patients become incontinent, unable to feed themselves and severely demented. Death follows within 10 years of the onset of symptoms.

In the early stages of the disease, there is a relatively selective loss of the GABA/enkephalin neurons in the striatum which project to the GPe. Later, all the medium spiny neurons of the striatum are affected and the pathology becomes widespread with the principal affected areas of the brain being the caudate, putamen, globus pallidus and cerebral cortex. It is believed that chorea is a result of basal ganglia deficit, whereas dementia is caused by cortical cell loss.

Paradoxically, despite the excess of involuntary movements, voluntary movements in patients with Huntington's disease are, like those of Parkinson's disease, slower than normal. Nevertheless, their movements are much more variable than those in patients with Parkinson's disease probably because of contamination by involuntary activity. The question arises as to whether it is possible, on the basis of our present models of the basal ganglia, to explain this strange combination of hyperkinesia (excess involuntary movement) and bradykinesia (slowness of movement). Thompson *et al.* [22] have suggested that the functional consequences of changes in activity of the direct and indirect pathways through the basal ganglia (see Fig. 1) are not equivalent. As discussed above, under-activity in the projection from subthalamic nucleus to the GPi (produced, in chorea, by excessive inhibition from the GPe) may play a crucial role in hyperkinesia. Perhaps under-activity in the direct pathway to the internal pallidal segment is important in producing bradykinesia. Such a theory would be consistent with results in Parkinson's disease. Lack of dopamine results in under-activity in the direct striatal projection to the GPi, and, via an opposite action on the indirect pathway, to excess excitatory output from the subthalamic nucleus. This would produce both bradykinesia and hypokinesia. In the mid-stages of Huntington's disease, when chorea is florid and all the cells of the striatum may be affected, a reduced output from the subthalamic nucleus would result in hyperkinesia, and a lack of activity in the striopallidal projection to the GPi would lead to bradykinesia. However, the theory is speculative.

Dystonia

Dystonia is a term used to describe twisted, sustained postures of the limbs, neck or trunk. In contrast to the forever changing, fleeting muscle contractions of chorea, dystonia describes a relatively fixed posture maintained by abnormal muscle activity. The condition is rare and in most incidences its cause is unknown. However, since similar clinical symptoms can be seen in patients with clear damage to the basal ganglia, it is usually thought that dystonia results from a basal ganglia deficit.

Little is known about the physiology of dystonia. The muscle spasms are characterized by co-contraction of antagonist muscles, rather than the more usual reciprocal pattern seen in many normal voluntary movements. Studies of spinal reflex pathways have shown a disorder of reciprocal inhibition in these patients which may contribute to the co-contracting activity [23]. Such a disorder of spinal mechanisms has been postulated to be due to abnormalities in the tonic descending control of spinal interneurons. Precisely how the basal ganglia might be involved in such tonic descending control is unknown, although, as suggested above for the postural difficulties of Parkinson's disease, they may result from the non-thalamic outputs of the basal ganglia to brainstem structures.

Conclusions

▶ The cerebral cortex is the main input to the basal ganglia and the prime output target. A small portion of the output also travels to brainstem structures. Within this cortico-basal ganglia-cortical loop, inputs for different cortical areas remain separate. The 'motor loop' from primary motor, and premotor and supplementary motor areas of cortex is one of the best studied.

▶ The 'direct' and 'indirect' pathways are the two major routes of information flow through the basal ganglia. Dopaminergic innervation from the substantia nigra pars compacta is inhibitory to neurones of the indirect pathway and excitatory to neurones of the direct pathway.

▶ The major output nuclei of the basal ganglia are the internal segment of the globus pallidus, and the substantia nigra pars reticulata. Cells in both these areas have a high tonic rate of discharge, and their output is inhibitory onto cells within the thalamus.

▶ Most theories of basal ganglia function assume that removal of tonic inhibitory output causes, or at least facilitates, movement. Increased inhibitory output may result in suppression of unwanted movement.

▶ Diseases of the basal ganglia produce either an excess or a paucity of movement. Three main conditions are recognized: Parkinson's disease, Huntingdon's disease and torsion dystonia.

► The most common disease of basal ganglia is Parkinson's disease. The major features are bradykinesia, tremor and rigidity, with postural difficulties becoming more apparent in the later stages of the disease. Lack of dopaminergic input from the substantia nigra pars compacta results in an increase in the final tonic inhibitory output of the internal glubus pallidus and the substantia nigra pars reticulata. In terms of basal ganglia theories this may interfere with the production of voluntary movement. New surgical approaches to the treatment of Parkinson's disease involve reducing this inhibitory output either by lesioning the subthalamic nucleus, or lesioning the internal segment of the globus pallidus.

References

1. Alexander, G.E. and Crutcher, M.D. (1990) Functional architecture of basal ganglia circuits: neural substrates of parallel processing. Trends Neurosci. **13**, 266–271

2. Smith, A.D. and Bolam, J.P. (1990) The neural network of the basal ganglia as revealed by the study of synaptic connections of identified neurones. Trends Neurosci. **13**, 259–265

3. Alexander, G.E. and Crutcher, M.D. (1990) Preparation for movement: neural representations of intended direction in three motor areas of the monkey. J. Neurophysiol. **64**, 133–150 (see also pp. 150–163 and 164–178)

4. Hoover, J.E. and Strick, P.L. (1993) Multiple output channels in the basal ganglia. Science **259**, 819–821

5. Graybiel, A.M. (1990) Neurotransmitters and neuromodulators in the basal ganglia. Trends Neurosci. **13**, 244–253

6. DeLong, M.R. and Georgopoulos, A.P. (1981) Motor functions of the basal ganglia. In: Handbook of Physiology (Brooks, V.B., ed.), Section 1, vol. 2, part 2, pp. 1017–1061, Williams and Wilkins, Baltimore

7. Crutcher, M.D. and Delong, M.R. (1984) Single cell studies of the primate putamen. Exp. Brain Res. **53**, 233–258

8. Chevalier, G. and Deniau, J.M. (1990) Disinhibition as a basic process in the expression of striatal function. Trends Neurosci. **13**, 277–280

9. Hikosaka, O. and Wurtz, R.H. (1983) Visual and oculomotor functions of monkey substantia nigra pars reticulata. Parts 1–4. J. Neurophysiol. **49**, 1232–1301

10. Mink, J.W. and Thach, W.T. (1991) Basal ganglia motor control. Parts 1, 2 and 3. J. Neurophysiol. **65**, 273–351

11. Brotchie, P., Iansek, R. and Horne, M.K. (1991) Motor function of the monkey globus pallidus. Papers 1 and 2. Brain **114**, 1667–1702

12. Romo, R. and Schultz, W. (1990) Dopamine neurones of the monkey midbrain: contigences of responses to active touch to self-initiated arm movement. J. Neurophysiol. **63**, 592–606 (See also following paper, pp. 607–624)

13. Filion, M. and Tremblay, L. (1991) Abnormal spontaneous activity of globus pallidus neurones in monkeys with MPTP induced parkinsonism. Brain Res. **547**, 142–151 (See also pp. 152–161)

14. Bergman, H., Wichmann, T. and DeLong, M.R. (1990) Reversal of experimental parkinsonism by lesions of the subthalamic nucleus. Science **249**, 1436–1438

15. Dick, J.P.R., Rothwell, J.C. and Day, B.L. (1989) The Bereitschaftspotential is abnormal in Parkinson's disease. Brain **112**, 233–244

16. Evarts, E.V., Teravainen, N.H. and Calne, D.B. (1981) Reaction time in Parkinson's disease. Brain **104**, 167–186

17. Anderson, M.E. and Horak, F.B. (1985) Influence of the globus pallidus on arm movement in monkeys. Parts 1, 2 and 3. J. Neurophysiol. **52**, 290–304 (see also pp. 305–322; vol. **54**, pp. 433–448)

18. Benecke, R., Rothwell, J.C., Dick, J.P.R. et al. (1987) Disturbance of sequential movements in patients with Parkinson's disease. Brain **110**, 361–379

19. Marsden, C.D. (1984) Origins of normal and pathological tremor. In: Movement Disorders: Tremor, (Findley, L.J. and Capildeo, R., eds.), pp. 37–84, Macmillan, London

20. Lamarre, Y. and Joffroy, A.J. (1979) Experimental tremor in monkey: activity of thalamic and precentral cortical neurones in the absence of peripheral feedback. Adv. Neurol. **24**, 109–122

21. Vidailhet, M., Rothwell, J.C., Thompson, P.D., Lees, A.J. and Marsden, C.D. (1992) The auditory startle response in the Steele–Richardson–Olszewski syndrome and Parkinson's disease. Brain **115**, 1181–1192

22. Thompson, P.D., Berardelli, A., Rothwell, J.C. et al. (1988) The co-existence of bradykinesia and chorea in Huntington's disease and its implications for theories of basal ganglia control of movement. Brain **111**, 223–244

23. Nakashima, K., Rothwell, J.C., Day, B.L., Thompson, P.D., Shannon, K. and Marsden, C.D. (1989) Reciprocal inhibition between forearm muscles in patients with writer's cramp and other occupational cramps, symptomatic hemidystonia and hemiparesis. Brain **112**, 681–697

3

The posterior parietal cortex, the cerebellum and the visual guidance of movement

John Stein
University Laboratory of Physiology, University of Oxford, Oxford, U.K.

Introduction

Over one-third of the human brain is devoted to the analysis of visual input. Hence vision plays a crucial role in the control not only of eye movements but also the majority of arm and body movements; and a high proportion of patients with brain damage suffer disordered visuomotor control, as do many children with developmental disorders. Moreover it is now a major aim of robotics research to develop useful visual guidance systems for these. It is clear therefore that a good understanding of the neurological mechanisms which underlie visuomotor control should provide theoretical, clinical and highly practical benefits. In this chapter I will consider the role of two of the most important structures which are implicated in the visual guidance of movement, namely the posterior parietal cortex and the cerebellum.

What and where visual pathways

The logical place to start to analyse the visual guidance of movement is at the output stages of the visual system. Over the last 20 years evidence has been accumulating that visual processing can be divided into a number of partially separate parallel pathways. These culminate in two main outflows, often known as the what and where outputs of the visual system [1]. Actually the 'where' pathway would be better described as the 'how' pathway because it is mainly concerned with guiding movement, as we shall see later. The two divisions are not entirely separate, however. There are numerous reciprocal cross-connections between them and also feedback from more specialized areas to the ones that project to them. The latter are particularly important for solving the 'binding problem'; identifying which of the separate specialized

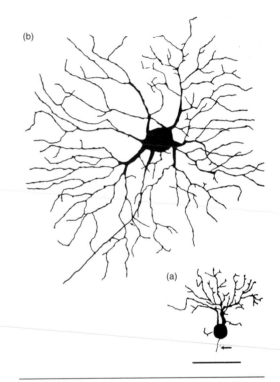

(b)

(a)

Fig. 1. (a) Parvo- and (b) magno-retinal ganglion cells
The axon is arrowed. Scale bar = 100 μmm.

operations being carried out by higher centres are dealing with the same object in the outside world. But it is still useful to divide the outputs of the visual system into two main pathways, because they serve rather different functions.

About 60% of the ganglion cells in the retina are small, parvocellular, neurons (Fig. 1) with 'sustained' responses, meaning that they are slowly adapting, so they continue to respond to a maintained visual stimulus. They signal the fine detail and colour of objects. Hence they provide the main signals for identifying objects for the what system. This stream

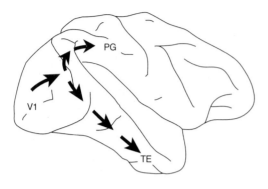

Fig. 2. The 'what?' stream projects to infero-temporal cortex area TE (Brodmann's area 21); the 'where?' stream to posterior parietal cortex (PPC) area PG (Brodmann's area 7a)

Posterior parietal cortex

The PPC is the archetypal cortical sensori-motor association area [2]. As shown in Fig. 3 it lies behind the primary somaesthetic area (Brodmann's areas 1, 2 and 3) and in front of prestriate cortex in the occipital lobe. Laterally it is bounded by the lateral (Sylvian) fissure; and medially it continues down to the cingulate cortex on the medial surface of the hemisphere. It contains superior and inferior parietal lob-ules. In monkeys the superior lobule consists of areas 5a and 5b and the inferior lobule, 7a and 7b; but in humans areas 5 and 7 both appear to lie in the superior parietal lobule and the infe-rior parietal lobule contains two new areas, 39 and 40, also known as the angular and supra-marginal gyri. Those on the left side are thought to be specialized to some extent for temporal processing, particularly of speech, whereas those on the right are more important for visuospatial function.

projects mainly ventrally and laterally into the inferotemporal cortex (Fig. 2); thus lesions there impair the ability to determine what an object is. In humans this is known as visual agnosia.

Some 10% of retinal ganglion cells are about three times larger, magnocellular or 'transient', neurons (Fig. 1). They respond pha-sically to the transient at the beginning and end of visual stimulation. So they signal the timing of visual events from which the motion of tar-gets may be derived for the where system to determine where targets are and how they are moving. They project mainly medially and dor-sally towards the superior temporal sulcus and posterior parietal cortex (PPC) as shown in Fig. 2. Since such phasic signals are needed for visuomotor control, PPC lesions disturb the visual guidance of eye and limb movements; and they interfere with how movements are carried out.

The PPC receives connections from all the areas surrounding it and from many distant ones as well (Fig. 3). Visual transient signals about the timing and motion of targets pass to the lateral side of the intraparietal sulcus (LIP) and 7a from the prestriate and middle temporal motion areas. Somaesthetic and proprioceptive signals about the current position and move-ments of the limbs pass from somaesthetic cor-tex just in front, to areas 5, 7b and the ventral intraparietal area (VIP). Area 7 also receives input from the vestibular and auditory cortex which lie laterally to it; and the whole of the PPC receives an important motivational input from the cingulate gyrus medially. Its main out-puts are to the frontal eye fields, the basal gan-glia, the pulvinar of the thalamus, the superior colliculus; and, in addition, it gives a very large projection to the cerebellum via the pontine nuclei. Since all these connections are reciprocal they serve as important inputs also.

The important features of the receptive field properties of PPC neurons are that they combine different sensory and motor inputs under the influence of the animal's sensory attention or motor intention. Thus they are much more active in response to a sensory stim-ulus when that stimulus is the subject of their attention or an intended movement. Most is known about the cells which respond to visual stimuli. Their receptive fields are usually large, often including the whole of one hemifield plus

▶ The visual system has what and where outputs for, respectively, identifying the detail and location of objects. The what out-put projects to the inferotemporal cortex and the where output to the posterior parietal cortex (PPC).
▶ The where output is used for visual guid-ance of eye and limb movements.

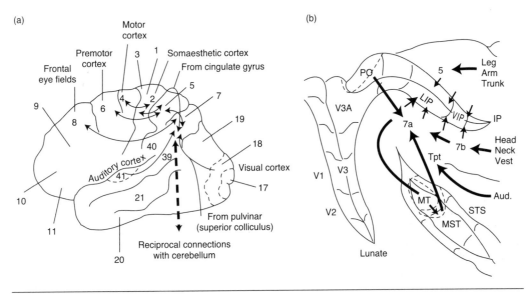

Fig. 3. (a) Connections of the PPC and (b) PPC subdivisions

(b) Abbreviations: V1, V2, V3, V3A, visual areas; PO, parieto-occipital junction; IP, intraparietal sulcus; LIP, lateral intraparietal area; VIP, ventral intraparietal area; 7a, 7b, and 5, Brodmann's areas; STS, superior temporal sulcus; MT, medial temporal area; MST, medial superior temporal area Tpt, parietotemporal area.

10 or more degrees of the ipsilateral field. Most do not respond to targets at the fovea, however; this is known as foveal sparing. As befits their transient input they are most sensitive to moving targets; and they are not interested in the form or colour of objects. They fire most vigorously when the animal is going to make an eye movement to an object within their receptive field, even if the target is extinguished by the time the animal begins to make the movement. In other words they can respond equally well to the memory of a target as to the target itself. It has been shown by replacing one target unexpectedly by another that PPC neuronal responses are determined by the animal's intended movement rather than what movement is actually made.

Many parietal neurons also receive non-retinal information about the position and movements of the eyes in the orbit. For example if the retinal location of a stimulus is kept constant, but the animal is required to look in different directions, their discharge for the same retinotopic stimulus is greatest for a particular direction of gaze, usually towards one side. So their overall discharge is an amalgam of the retinal position of the target, the position of the eyes and the animal's intended movement. Zipser and Andersen developed a neural network model of these features which shows how such neurons with large receptive fields and weak eye position signals could together generate a representation of the position of objects in the outside world independent of where the eyes are pointing [3]. This network converts the coordinate system for locating objects from a retinotopic one in which their positions move each time the eyes do, into an egocentric one in which the location of a target is represented with respect to the centre of the body, the egocentre.

It is often assumed that in order to perform the wide variety of such coordinate transformations which have to be made, the PPC converts all the sensory and motor coordinate systems into a common currency, so as to represent the external world in the form of a general purpose topographical map of egocentric space. But no such common space map has ever been found. Zipser and Andersen's neural network simulation did not generate a topographical map; instead it produced a distributed 'look up table' of the located objects. This is analogous to the gazetteer at the back of an atlas; in this the location of places is given by their map references. Such coordinates can be used without a map. They are really rules which indicate how to get to each place. In the same way the PPC probably does not form a topographical map of the outside world; there is no point to point correspondence between points in the PPC and locations in the external world [4]. Instead it contains a representation of the rules or algorithms which must be employed to get from a to b. These are required to translate between different sensory reference frames or from sensory to motor coordinate systems; the one that is chosen seems to depend on the direction of attention or what movements are intended. The neural embodiment of each of these algorithms appears to be distributed over the whole PPC, so that small lesions attenuate them all rather than eliminating a single one. Thus the PPC employs a large number of different reference frames, one for each and every sensory and sensorimotor conversion that is needed. Hence eye movements are controlled largely retinotopically, but calibrated by eye position information; arm movements are made in a coordinate system centred on the shoulder; finger movements are referenced to the centre of the hand; and so on.

The effects of PPC lesions support the idea that its function is to transform between different sensory and motor coordinate systems according to where and when the subject wishes to direct attention or movements. The classic sign of PPC lesions is contralateral neglect, failure to direct attention to the side contralateral to the lesion. Hence patients leave out contralateral details when copying pictures, as shown in Fig. 4, or when drawing from memory. Their main difficulty may not be inability to direct their attention to the contralateral side, but rather inability to disengage their attention from the ipsilateral side, perhaps because impulses passing across the corpus callosum from objects of potential interest on the contralateral side fail to inhibit attentional mechanisms on the good side.

The nature of the coordinate system of the space which is neglected in parietal neglect patients is clearly of great interest. If the PPC is involved in coordinate transformations which are primarily designed for motor control one would expect that its representation of space would not move around each time the eyes or

limbs do. In other words it should be related to a fixed point such as the centre of the body, the so-called egocentre. But the situation turns out to be more complicated than this. First, as described earlier the particular coordinate system employed varies with the nature of the movement; so, for example, eye movements are mainly encoded in retinotopic coordinates centred on the fovea; whereas arm movements appear to be centred on the shoulder; and head and body movements are referenced to the egocentre. Memorized or imagined movements are also related to the patient's egocentre. In an experiment which has justly become famous Edoardo Bisiach asked neglect patients to imagine entering the Piazza del Duomo in Milan from one end and to describe the buildings they saw. He found that they only reported the buildings on the right of the square. But when they were asked to imagine entering from the other end of the square they changed to neglecting the buildings they had previously reported, and now they read out the ones that they had previously neglected. So clearly somewhere they had intact memories of all the buildings; it was the patients' ability to consciously relate the locations of these buildings to their own bodies which was impaired.

In addition, however, whether or not visual features are treated as separate or components of a single object is important. The left side of objects is neglected. If there are two separate objects the left sides of both are neglected. Whether it is the left half of a picture that is neglected or the left half of two objects in the picture depends upon how separate the two objects are. And the left side of objects may be neglected irrespective of whether they are situated on the patient's left or right side; i.e. neglect is often object-centred rather than egocentred. Nevertheless it is the left side of the object in relation to the patient that is neglected, but that could be on the right of the patient's egocentre.

PPC lesions usually also impair the guidance of movement; the most obvious effects are on eye movements. The eyes fail to follow a moving target smoothly; instead they make a series of steps (Fig. 5). The worst effects are usually for the direction ipsilateral to the lesion. This may be because when tracking a moving target the eyes tend to lag behind it. Because contralateral neglect tends to be object-centred, this means that the eyes tend to be pointed to

Model   Patient's copy

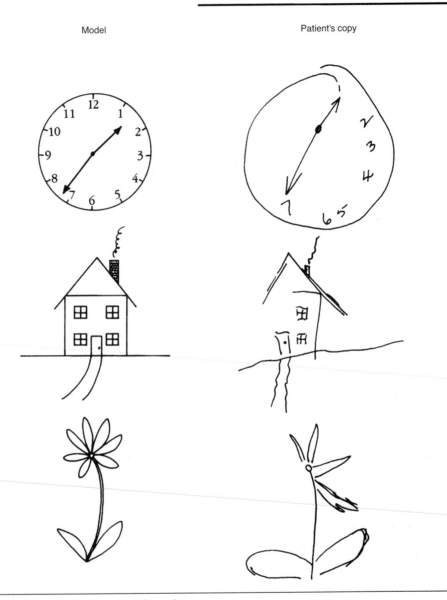

Fig. 4. Examples of left neglect

the contralateral, neglected, side of the target when it is going towards the same side as the lesion but not when it is going in the opposite direction. In contrast saccades to the contralateral side are the most impaired. Contralateral targets tend to be neglected, so the patients do not look towards them; and also saccades made towards the contralateral side are often hypometric, falling short of their target, so that two or more may be required before a target on that side is foveated.

PPC lesions also severely impair binocular, vergence, eye movement control, so that diplopia and oscillopsia (apparent movement of the visual world) are quite common. The combination of neglect and oscillopsia due to unstable binocular control causes many patients with PPC lesions to find reading very difficult (neglect dyslexia). Some developmental dyslexics seem to have similar, though milder, problems; the visual confusion engendered by their

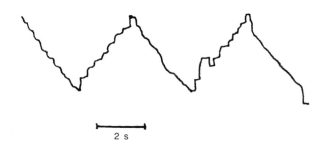

2 s

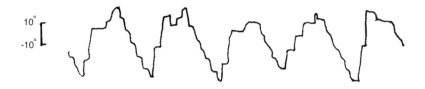

10°
-10°

Saccadic intrusions during smooth pursuit in patient with PPC lesion

Fig. 5. Effect of right PPC lesion on smooth pursuit eye movements
Patient attempting to track a triangle wave: right, positive; left, negative. Note breakdown to saccadic steps particularly for rightwards and faster movements (lower trace).

oculomotor and perceptual instability probably contributes to their reading difficulties [5].

Other visually guided movements are also often impaired by PPC lesions. Pointing at targets, reaching out for things, and navigating around the world are all inaccurate, so that damage to this part of the cortex is highly disabling.

In summary, therefore, the PPC seems to contain a distributed neural network which embodies instructions for converting between different sensory and motor reference frames. The function which is traditionally ascribed to the PPC is to maintain a representation of the position of targets in the outside world and of the parts of the body, i.e. to build up a map of egocentric space. But the way in which the PPC locates objects in the outside world seems not to require the drawing of a topographic map of 'real' space there. Instead it seems to consist of a distributed neural network which implements instructions which specify how to aim attention, eyes, body or limbs at targets in the outside world [4]. Clearly the only reason for localizing targets is to direct attention or move-

ments towards them; and this seems to be what the PPC is for.

▶ The PPC maintains a representation of the position of objects in the outside world and of parts of the body.
▶ The PPC comprises a neural network providing instructions of how to aim attention, eyes, body or limbs at targets in the outside world.
▶ The PPC projects to four main motor areas, (1) the prefrontal cortex and frontal eye fields, (2) the basal ganglia, (3) the superior colliculus and (4) the cerebellum.

Visuomotor projections

The neuroanatomical way to continue our investigation of the visual guidance of movement is to consider the pathways which run from the PPC to the motor areas of the brain. There are four main outputs which we must

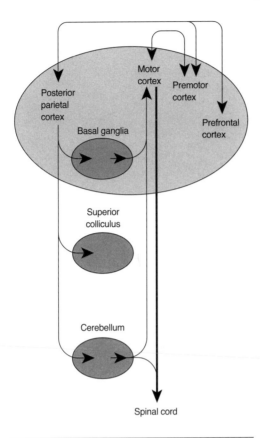

Fig. 6. The four main outputs of the PPC

consider (Fig. 6). These are the intracortical projection from PPC to the prefrontal cortex and frontal eye fields via the superior longitudinal fasciculus, and the three subcortical pathways which link visual with motor areas, via the basal ganglia, the superior colliculus and cerebellum.

The connections to the frontal cortex and to the basal ganglia are probably relatively unimportant for guiding movements visually. Lesions in either pathway have little effect on the accuracy or speed of visually guided movements. If all the corticocortical fibres connecting the PPC with the frontal cortex are cut in monkeys, the animals' ability to pick up food from a moving turntable is hardly altered. Likewise it is well known that visually guided movements often survive basal ganglia damage. Striking is the contrast between parkinsonian patients' relatively fluent visually guided move-

ments and their inability to produce spontaneous movements. They can often match their steps to marks painted on the floor, or catch a ball thrown towards them; but they find it much more difficult to throw it back again or to start walking with no marks to aim for. Similarly although lesions of the superior colliculus disturb the direction of saccadic eye movements the effects are short lived unless the frontal eye fields or PPC are lesioned at the same time, and they have little effect on smooth pursuit or limb movements.

In contrast inactivation of the output of the cerebellum often has a decimating effect on the accuracy of visually guided movements of either eyes or limbs (Fig. 7a); and, as Gordon Holmes was one of the first to point out, this is permanent if a large lesion is made.

The cerebellar cortex receives two very different kinds of input: mossy and climbing fibres. It has a fundamentally simple three-layered geometric structure based on the Purkinje cell (P cell). It is like a matrix in its uniform regularity (Fig. 8). It seems likely therefore that

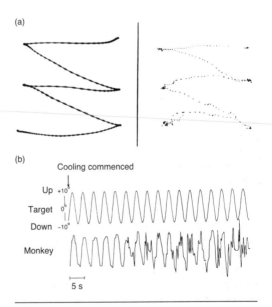

Fig. 7. (a) Incoordination of right arm tracking a visual target in a Holme's patient with right cerebellar lesion compared with the unaffected left arm (left-hand trace) and (b) the effect of inactivating dentate nucleus on a monkey tracking a visual target with a hand-held lever

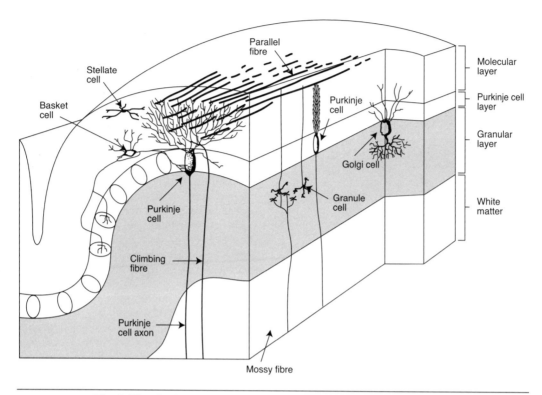

Fig. 8. Histological structure of the cerebellar cortex

every part of the cerebellar cortex performs the same basic processing operation. In the deepest, granule cell, layer the granule cells receive the mossy fibre input via their glomerular dendrites. There are an astronomical number of these small cells, estimated at 10^{11}. Their axons are directed towards the surface of the folium past the P cell bodies; and there in the most superficial, parallel fibre, or molecular, layer they divide in a T junction to form the parallel fibres. These then run parallel to the surface through the flattened dendritic trees of the P cells which are situated at right angles to the surface of the folium. Some 200 000 pass through the dendritic tree of each P cell, each making one synapse with it. Each parallel fibre is from 3 to 6 mm long and can therefore synapse with up to 250 P cells. Probably less than 0.5% (1000) of its complement of parallel fibres have to be activated more or less simultaneously to excite 'simple' spikes from the P cells (Fig. 9b).

Visual timing and motion signals are passed from the prestriate and PPC via the dorsolateral pontine nuclei as mossy fibre inputs;

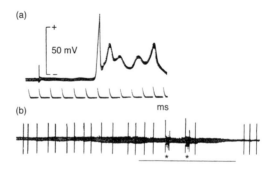

Fig. 9. (a) Complex spike (intracellular recording) and (b) simple spikes (extracellular recording)

(b) Two complex spikes (marked with *) elicited by passive paw movement inhibit simple spike activity.

these reach most parts of the cerebellar cortex [6]. Those from the superior colliculus pass via a slightly different region of the pontine nuclei. Simple spike activity in response to visual stimuli can therefore be recorded from most parts of the cerebellar cortex; but there are particularly dense inputs to the posterior vermis and the extreme lateral cortex. In primates these regions are the uvula medially and the dorsal paraflocculus laterally. The latter is not part of the vestibular flocculus as used to be thought; it receives dense visual but little vestibular input.

The climbing fibre input to P cells could not be more different. All climbing fibres are axons of neurons situated in the inferior olive (IO). Each P cell receives just one; it climbs around its dendrites making up to 500 synapses. Each inferior olivary axon divides well below the cortical surface to provide climbing fibres to up to 10 widely separated P cells. Their discharge excites a climbing fibre or 'complex spike' in each of the recipient P cells (Fig. 9a). Typically IO neurons discharge only once or twice a second. They respond to sensory events

(a)

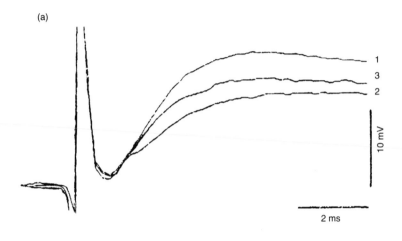

(b)

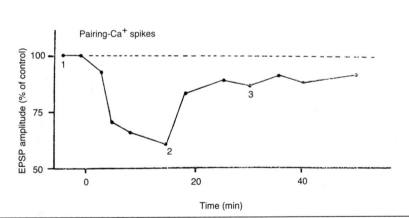

Fig. 10. Long-term depression
Patient attempting to track a triangle wave: right, positive; left, negative. Note breakdown to saccadic steps particularly for rightwards and faster movements (lower trace).

in the outside world, such as touching the skin (exafference), rather than to the sensory consequences of one's own movements (reafference). Their responses are therefore inhibited if a stimulus is the expected consequence of a movement, e.g. the touch down when walking.

The climbing fibre discharge consists of a profound Na depolarization of the P cell, lasting for over 10 ms. On the depolarized plateau are superimposed two to five high-threshold Ca spikelets. Each complex spike is succeeded by a pause in simple spike activity for about 10 ms, and this is often followed by some hundreds of ms or so of further inhibition of simple spike activity (Fig. 9b). It is now clear that over an even longer time span, of hours or days after climbing fibre activity, the parallel fibre synapses which happened to be active when it fired continue to be depressed. This is known as long-term depression (LTD) [7] (Fig. 10). Probably the influx of Ca caused by the complex spikelets down-regulates P-cell glutamate receptors via a G-protein-dependent kinase. However, when a P cell is not depolarized sufficiently to switch on the high-threshold Ca conductance, which is what climbing fibre discharges achieve, a succession of simple spike depolarizations can lead to the opposite effect, i.e. long-term potentiation (LTP), of subsequent parallel fibre inputs, rather than LTD. These opposing mechanisms probably form the basis of cerebellar 'learning'.

Some IO cells supplying climbing fibres to the flocculus receive their visual input from an area which lies in front of the superior colliculus, the pretectal area; and this in turn is supplied by its own specialized visual pathway, the accessory optic tract system. Their response to external sensory events suggests that in general climbing fibre discharges may indicate when reflex or semiautomatic motor systems are not quite working properly. So during vestibulo-ocular or smooth pursuit eye movements a potent stimulus is 'retinal slip', when the velocity of the eyes does not quite match that of the target properly, so the target is tending to slip off the fovea. Thus climbing fibres may discharge when the actual sensory consequences of a movement are different from those which were intended. They are often referred to as error detectors; but this description is somewhat misleading. Since climbing fibres only discharge about once per second they can only signal that an unexpected event has occurred, not

its size or timing. At first sight such an error signal does not seem ideal for motor learning, because its information content is too low; it is too 'low quality'. But precise information is being supplied all the time by the mossy fibre system. The problem is to decide what are error signals and what are normal sensory consequences of a movement. Perhaps this is the main function of the climbing fibres, to identify which mossy fibre inputs denote motor error, and to distinguish these from signals about the predictable consequences of a movement (reafference).

> The cerebellum is closely involved in the visuo-motor control of eye and limb movements; the most important regions, in primates, are the posterior vermis and extreme lateral cortex, the paraflocculus.
> The cerebellum has two main types of input, mossy and climbing fibres, which respectively produce 'simple' and 'complex' spikes in cerebellar cortical output Purkinje cells. Mossy fibre inputs from the prestriate cortex and PPC signal visual timing and motion. The climbing fibres are thought to signal when the sensory consequences of movement differ from those intended; they signal unexpected events or errors.

The cerebellum as a metasystem

An important feature of the anatomical connections of the cerebellum is that it does not lie on any of the direct pathways linking sensory with motor centres [8]. For example the basic circuit underlying the vestibulo-ocular reflex is a three-neuron arc (Fig. 11). The semicircular canals project to the vestibular nuclei; vestibular axons then run in the medial longitudinal fasciculus to supply the motoneurons controlling the external ocular muscles. Thus if the right horizontal canal is stimulated by rightwards movements of the head, after a latency of only 10 ms the left lateral rectus and the right medial rectus muscles contract, causing the eyes to move to the left, and thus to compensate for the head movement, so the gaze remains pointing straight ahead. The cerebellum has no part to play in this direct pathway. However, it does receive mossy fibre input from all three sites,

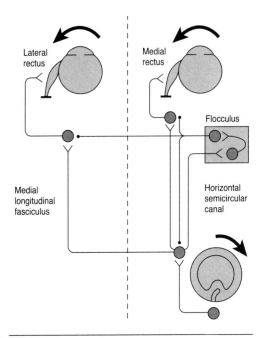

Fig. 11. Basic wiring diagram for VOR

—<, excitatory synapse; —•, inhibitory synapse. Note that the connections with the flocculus lie in parallel to the direct reflex pathway, for calibrating it.

red nuclei and the rubrospinal tract directly to the spinal cord, particularly supplying motoneurons controlling distal extensor muscles. In addition it projects via VL, motor cortex and the corticospinal tract to distal flexor muscles of the limbs (Fig. 12). The medial cerebellar cortex receives from the vestibular system and spinocerebellar tracts and projects via the fastigial nucleus to the vestibular system and adjacent reticular formation, thence to proximal limb and postural musculature. So the medial division of the cerebellum is more concerned with postural and reflex control, and the intermediate cerebellum more with distal musculature for voluntary control. The lateral cerebellum is by far the largest part in humans; relative to its size in lower animals it has grown even larger than the cerebral cortex. Yet its function remains to a large extent a mystery.

Stimulation, recording and observing the effects of lesions have been the main techniques employed for trying to understand the functions of different parts of the nervous system. Stimulation of the cerebellum has not proved very illuminating, however; mainly because the only output of the cerebellar cortex, the P cell, is inhibitory on its target nuclear cells. Hence stimulating the cerebellar cortex can arrest movements that are in progress; but this does not tell us much about how it helps to control them.

▶ The uniform geometric structure of the cerebellar cortex suggests a generalized processing function.
▶ The cerebellum acts as a supervisor or metasystem; it operates in parallel to other motor circuits and automates, calibrates and optimizes them, e.g. adjusts parameters of reflexes such as VOR (vestibulo-ocular reflex).
▶ The cerebellum is organized into longitudinal and functional sub-divisions and separate output nuclei and connections to other motor systems. The medial division of the cerebellum is mainly concerned with postural and reflex control, the intermediate division with distal muscles for voluntary control. The function of the large lateral division (hemispheres) is uncertain.

the labyrinth, the vestibular and oculomotor nuclei, and it projects inhibitory synapses back to them. Thus it forms a side pathway to the basic reflex circuitry. Its function seems to be to adjust the parameters of the reflex, to calibrate it to suit different circumstances. This seems to be the general rule; the cerebellum operates in parallel to other circuits in order to automate, calibrate and optimize them; hence it can be described as a supervisor or metasystem.

The output of the cerebellum passes via the deep cerebellar nuclei, of which there are three on each side: the lateral (dentate), intermediate (interpositus) and medial (fastigial) nuclei. These three define three distinct longitudinal, and functional, subdivisions. The lateral cerebellar cortex receives mainly from the cerebral cortex and projects via the dentate nucleus and ventralis lateralis (VL) nucleus of the thalamus mainly back to the premotor cortex (PMC; Fig. 12). The interpositus nucleus receives from the intermediate cerebellar cortex which in turn receives from the motor cortex and spinocerebellar tracts. It projects via the interpositus and

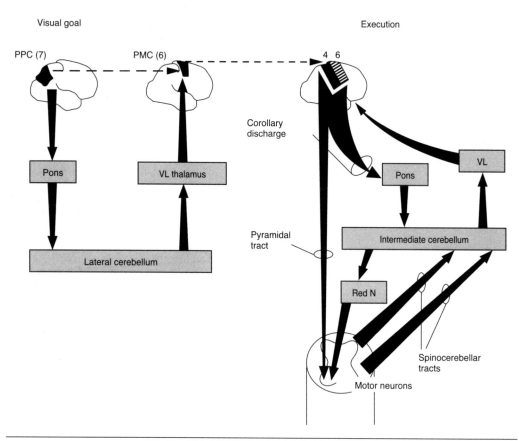

Fig. 12. Cerebellum as a metasystem
Lateral cerebellum operates in parallel with the direct cortical pathway which links PPC to premotor cortex; intermediate cerebellum works in parallel with the cortico-spinal tract.

Effects of lesions

Most of our understanding of the cerebellum has come from studying lesions in man. Although it seems to be less vulnerable to disease than for example the basal ganglia, trauma, tumours, strokes, multiple sclerosis and congenital diseases all afflict it, and it is probably responsible for familial and senile tremors. From the earliest descriptions of Luciani and Flourens it has been clear that cerebellar lesions do not cause paralysis; they do not prevent movements taking place. Instead patients become uncoordinated, and their movements lose their smoothness, speed and skill. Cerebellar patients have consciously to concentrate closely on every movement they make; their actions are no longer automatic. Gordon Holmes described three cardinal signs of cerebellar disease; hypotonia, postural ataxia and intention tremor [9]. Of these hypotonia is the least reliable; it is probably the result of incoordinated contraction of individual motor units in the muscles. Postural ataxia is inability to maintain a stable posture. Particularly when their eyes are closed, the patients sway around, become increasingly unstable and soon fall over. They stagger from side to side when walking. Intention tremor is ataxia of voluntary movement. On being asked to touch the examiner's finger the patient overshoots, overcorrects again and again; and has the same problems when attempting to touch his own nose.

We have to admit, however, that we still do not know precisely what the basic processing function of the cerebellum is, by which it achieves coordination of movement. The uniform geometric structure of the cerebellar cortex strongly suggests that it provides a generalized processing function which is applied to different parts of the body by the different connections of each region. That is why postural ataxia is caused by lesions of the midline (vermal) cerebellum; whereas limb ataxia, intention tremor, follows damage to the cerebellar hemispheres. But we are still not quite sure what the processing function is.

Recording in trained animals

When techniques for recording from awake animals trained to perform particular movements were introduced in the early 1970s, many of us thought that the true function of the cerebellum would at last be revealed. However, so far the results of these experiments have mostly been rather disappointing; one cannot honestly say that they have revealed much that we didn't know already from anatomical or lesion experiments. By means of recording we have been able to show that wide areas of the cerebellar cortex do indeed receive visual input and that this signals mainly the rate and direction of motion of targets, as expected from recording in the prestriate and posterior parietal areas and in the pontine nuclei. The discharge of many P cells in intermediate and lateral cerebellar cortex precedes movements. In the cortex signals coding the position, velocity or acceleration of the limbs can be recorded; and also one can record simple spike activity which is quantitatively related to the difference between the desired and actual position of the limbs. In other words the quantitatively accurate error signals which are needed for feedback control are supplied to the cerebellum by the mossy fibres, and coded in Purkinje cell discharge of simple spikes. In the cerebellar nuclei responses are more complex; probably they are related to the coordination of several joints. In the interpositus nucleus control of precision finger movements seems to be particularly important, whereas in the dentate signals relating to the planning and adaptation of limb movements are found.

However, none of these results has told us what the basic processing function of the cerebellar cortex really is. The striking advances have come from biophysical and pharmacological studies; these have led to much greater understanding of the ionic currents underlying simple and complex spikes in P cells and how these relate to long-term depression and potentiation (LTD and LTP), hence to possible learning functions of the cerebellum.

Calibration of feedforward control

To gain a greater understanding of the function of the cerebellum researchers have turned to recent advances in control system engineering. Many people implicitly assume that negative feedback control is the 'ideal' model we should use to understand the neural control of movement. It is true that servomechanisms have the great advantage that they are potentially very accurate; but they have one grave disadvantage. They are very susceptible to time delays. If the lag between deviations in their output and feedback of these to the controller is more than one-tenth of movement time negative feedback controllers tend to become destructively unstable. But visual feedback may take 100–200 ms to be processed. Hence any movement taking a shorter time than about 1 s would very likely be highly unstable if controlled by continuous negative feedback. Yet most of our movements actually take no more than about one-third of a second. Hence they are most unlikely to be guided by a negative feedback controller. They probably employ mainly feedforward control with feedback only switching in intermittently for error correction.

Feedforward control has the great advantage that it is not affected by time delays, because the control signal passes directly to the actuator. However, it suffers from a potentially equally disastrous disadvantage, namely inaccuracy. Only if the feedforward control programme is completely correctly calibrated will the system perform as desired. This requires that the outcome of each possible movement can be predicted ahead of time. Then the feedforward controller can be preloaded with the required program calibrated to achieve exactly the desired outcome.

The rest of this chapter will therefore be devoted to showing that such calibration is the general function of the cerebellum. I will describe some examples for which the calibration role has been worked out in some detail.

These will show how the wide variety of functions that have been suggested for the cerebellum all reduce to the single, simple, idea that it is a motor predictor for calibrating feedforward programs.

VOR adaptation

We will first consider in greater detail the role of the cerebellum in adaptation of the vestibulo-ocular reflex (VOR). It is now clear that one function of the flocculus is to calibrate the quantitative parameters of this feedforward reflex. As shown in Fig. 11 the basic circuitry of the VOR provides no feedback pathway. Yet the exact relationship between the number of impulses emitted from the semicircular canals following a head movement and the number of impulses required in the eye muscle motor neurons to achieve an exactly compensating eye movement is not fixed and immutable. It changes greatly over time because of the growth of the head and eyes, changing optical factors, etc, etc. So the VOR has to be continually recalibrated. Adaptation experiments have shown that the cerebellar flocculus is essential for such recalibration. If you wear reversing spectacles for a few days, vestibular eye movements adapt

to compensate, and the VOR can be made to reverse in direction (Fig. 13). After lesions of the cerebellar flocculus the VOR will not adapt in this way, however.

When the VOR is miscalibrated just after putting on reversing spectacles, the reflex no longer manages to keep targets on the fovea; they progressively slip further and further off it. The quantitative size of this slip is signalled to the flocculus by mossy fibres; the fact that this is unexpected slip rather than optic flow caused by your own eye movements, is signalled by climbing fibre discharges. The flocculus then adjusts the parameters of the VOR pathway to reverse its direction of action and thus avoid retinal slip. Hence if the flocculus is damaged the reflex cannot adapt to the new situation. Ito and Miles recorded floccular neurons before and after such adaptation, and showed that their discharge alters as would be expected if they play a crucial part in this kind of motor learning. These two groups interpret their results rather differently, however. Ito suggests that long-term changes only occur in the flocculus, whereas Miles believes that they occur both in the flocculus and the vestibular nuclei. But the fundamental point is the same; the flocculus is essential for recalibrating the VOR to adapt to changed optical conditions.

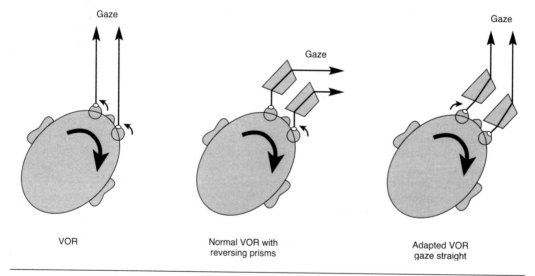

VOR

Normal VOR with reversing prisms

Adapted VOR gaze straight

Fig. 13. Adaptation of the vestibulo-ocular reflex (VOR)
(a) When head turns right, eyes turn left, so gaze remains straight ahead. (b) With reversing prisms if eyes turn left gaze points right. (c) After adaptation eyes now turn in same direction as head; so after reversal by prisms gaze points straight ahead again.

One way of describing these phenomena is to say that the cerebellum comes to be able to predict the bad sensory consequences of the unadapted VOR in the presence of reversing spectacles, hence to change its parameters to improve them.

Nictitating membrane reflex (NMR) conditioning

Another simple example of reflex adaptation is conditioning of the nictitating membrane reflex (NMR). This is another feedforward reflex; its conditioning also requires prediction. The nictitating membrane is the third eyelid that rabbits possess, which moves across when the eye retracts for protection if the cornea or surrounding skin is stimulated. If a stimulus to the cornea (the normal unconditioned stimulus, US) is preceded by a flash of light (the conditioning stimulus, CS) for 100 or so pairings the flash of light alone will begin to evoke the eyelid response; the reflex has become conditioned. This conditioning survives ablation of the whole neocortex and hippocampus. However, if a small region of anterior cerebellar cortex, paravermal lobule VI, is removed on one side the conditioned reflex on that side disappears. But the normal unconditioned response to the air puff remains intact. Furthermore it will now require several thousand pairings to recondition the reflex on that side and even this weak response disappears if the ablation is widened to include parts of lobule VII as well.

The precise area of the cerebellar cortex which is responsible for conditioning the NMR is determined by the topography of its climbing fibre input. The region of the IO which receives from the area around the eye projects climbing fibres to this crucial part of the cerebellar cortex. Thus the normal unconditioned stimulus for the reflex specifies the area of cortex which will mediate conditioning. This makes good sense because the IO climbing fibre system preserves body topography whereas the mossy fibre/parallel fibre system does not. During conditioning, the climbing fibres which project to paravermal VI are excited, and probably these reduce the efficacy with which concurrent visually driven parallel fibres excite those particular P cells (LTD see Fig. 14). Therefore these P cells no longer inhibit their target neurons in the interpositus nucleus, and so the

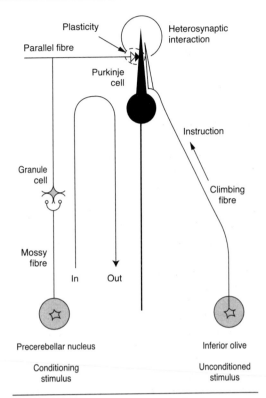

Fig. 14. Conditioning the nictitating membrane reflex (NMR)

Climbing fibres signal the normal, unconditioned, cutaneous stimulus for the reflex; parallel fibres deliver conditioning visual stimulus. Heterosynaptic interaction between climbing and parallel fibre inputs depresses specific synapses; this allows nuclear cells to respond to conditioning stimulus even when climbing fibres do not fire.

visual conditioning stimulus can elicit the reflex.

Calibration as prediction

Conditioning the NMR is a simple experimental paradigm in which a stimulus comes to predict that a particular motor response is going to be required. Soon the predictive stimulus alone is enough to provoke the motor response. In fact the calibration of all feedforward control processes can be seen as predictive in this way. In order to work properly all feedforward controllers have to be loaded with a program which is properly calibrated for the task in hand. This calibration can only be correct if it can draw on a precise prediction of what the sensory consequences of the movement will be.

The next example of how the cerebellum calibrates feedforward processes is the way in which it uses motion information provided by the visual system to program movements. When tracking a moving target whose trajectory is not entirely predictable we resort to making a series of intermittent steps rather than a smooth continuous movement. The advantage of this strategy is that it combines the virtues of both feedforward and feedback control. Each intermittent movement consists of a negative feedback component equal in size to the current error to compensate for it, and a second component which is calculated to allow for the continued movement of the target. The latter incorporates visual motion information about the speed with which the target is moving; this is used to predict where the target will be at the end of the forthcoming movement in order to program it to be the right size to catch up with the target. If both components are computed accurately the next movement lands precisely on target (Fig. 15).

Neurons in the dorsal paraflocculus receive signals about the rate and direction of moving targets. If the nuclear target of the dorsal paraflocculus, the ventral dentate, is inactivated by cooling or local anaesthetic in animals trained to track moving targets, the animals' tracking becomes more intermittent and jerky and much less accurate, as demonstrated in Fig. 7. Whereas before inactivation both current error and target velocity are good predictors of the size of the next movement, i.e. they are used to compute the correct amplitude for the movement, during inactivation movement amplitude is no longer adjusted to compensate for the speed with which the target is moving. In other words the animal is no longer able to use the velocity of the target to predict where it will be at the end of the next movement and to scale the size of the next movement accordingly.

> ▶ Principles of control systems engineering suggest that most visually guided movements are regulated by feedforward rather than negative feedback control.

> ▶ The cerebellum is thought to act as a motor predictor for calibrating feedforward programs.
> ▶ Examples of the cerebellum's (re)calibration function are adaptation of the VOR to changed optical conditions and conditioning of the nictating membrane reflex (NMR). The process of (re)calibration or adaptation is probably based on the long-term depression (LTD) and long-term potentiation (LTP) of granule cell parallel fibre inputs to Purkinje cells by parallel fibre–climbing fibre interactions; climbing fibre complex spike activity may retrain the simple spike activity of Purkinje cells.
> ▶ During calibration of feedforward reflex or voluntary processes the climbing fibres may report when something unexpected happens in the outside world and the concurrent Purkinje cell simple spike activity provides the quantitative detail required to correct the movement on subsequent occasions; combining parallel and climbing fibre discharges to set the activity level of Purkinje cells to calibrate movements may be the fundamental processing operation of the cerebellar cortex.

Visuomotor adaptation

The most direct way to show that the cerebellum is concerned with calibrating feedforward control processes is to test its function during adaptation since this is when recalibration will be most required. In the same way that the cerebellum is essential for adapting the VOR to reversing prisms, it is now known to be required for adapting reaching movements for the deviation of gaze that occurs if prisms are placed in front of the eyes. If subjects view through prisms, the visual axes are deviated; and they initially misaim at targets. After a few trials the visuomotor system adapts to the new visual situation and aiming returns to being on target. If the prisms are then removed misaiming occurs in the opposite direction for a few trials until readaptation occurs. But if the lateral cerebellum, including the dorsal paraflocculus, is removed in animals or damaged in humans such adaptation no longer occurs.

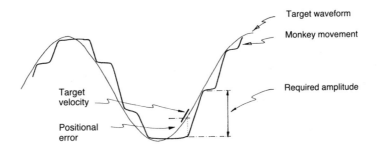

Fig. 15. Prediction of where target will be at end of a movement

To hit target, required amplitude of monkey's next movement must equal the motion of the target (target velocity × duration of the movement) + current positional error.

Similar adaptation can be established in animals trained to track a moving target with a lever if the amplitude of the lever movement required to track the target, i.e. the gain of the system, is altered. Monkeys cannot adapt to this gain change if the dentate nucleus is inactivated. During adaptation to changes in loading of the lever simple spike discharges corresponding to the inaccurate movements increase, and then as adaptation occurs they decrease again when the movements are accurate again. This change is accompanied by increases in climbing fibre responses; but it has proved difficult to show, as one would like, that this occurs in the same cells whose simple spike activity decreases during adaptation. Nevertheless these findings suggest that the complex spike activity may be retraining the simple spike activity of P cells. However, what the stimulus for the climbing fibre activity is under these circumstances is not yet known.

All these examples suggest that the cerebellum is probably involved in calibrating feedforward processes, whether reflex or voluntary. The climbing fibres probably report when something unexpected happens in the outside world and the simple spike activity occurring at the same time provides the quantitative information necessary to correct the movement on subsequent occasions. So the fundamental processing operation of the cerebellar cortex which we have all been looking for, may be to combine climbing and parallel fibre discharges to set the level of activity of P cells in order to calibrate movements precisely.

Internal models

To further understand how the cerebellum may calibrate feedforward control processes we really need to develop computer simulations of them, because the very basic models which we use implicitly when designing experiments, such as negative feedback or simple feedforward systems, do not capture the complexity of most real motor control situations. A useful way of conceptualizing the control problems is to consider the cerebellar cortex as laying down 'internal models' of the movements to be performed. The feedforward control signal is a program which has to be assembled and correctly calibrated before it can be used. A convenient way of generating such a program is to set up an internal model of the required movement which can then be played out when required.

Two rather different kinds of simulation of these internal representations have been developed by control theorists. An 'inverse' model represents the sequence of signals which will cause the controlled object to produce a desired movement. It is said to be the inverse of the controlled object because if it is correctly formulated, on being operated on by the controlled object, it will produce precisely the required output. Such inverse filters are popular with control engineers because they can be designed with mathematical precision to perform to any desired specification of accuracy. But it is very difficult to design them to be able to adapt to changing conditions; yet such plasticity is an essential feature of neurological control systems. Inverse filters are only useful

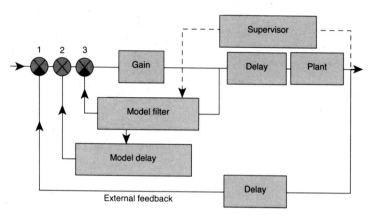

Analytic simulation: Smith predictor

Fig. 16. Smith predictor hypothesis

Cerebellum may hold a 'model' of the moving limb ('plant'), simulated here as a filter, and also a model of the time delay taken of the external feedback pathway for sensory signals about the outcome of a movement to return, so that it can delay output of the model to compare with what actually happened. It also acts as a 'supervisor' using the external feedback to optimize the models.

when they are perfectly calibrated. Unless they are that accurate they tend to be dangerous. So just when they are most required, during adaptation to new conditions, they cannot be used until they have been recalibrated.

The second kind of internal representation suggested for programming movements is a 'forward' model. Here the model is a neural replica of the required movement, rather than its inverse. So its output can be described as a prediction of the outcome of the desired movement. Since only our senses can tell us about this outcome, i.e. how well the movement was performed, the output of the model must take the form of a prediction of the sensory consequences of the movement. We saw earlier how such predictions contribute to programming movements. But the output of such a forward model cannot be used to control the limbs directly, because it is expressed in terms of the sensory consequences of the movement rather than specifying the signals required to actually drive the muscles to make it. The way round this problem is to put the forward model in an internal feedback loop. Then its output can be compared with the signal commanding the desired movement and the difference becomes the 'inverse' signal which is required for actually contracting muscles [10].

There are many advantages to this approach, and many people now believe that the cerebellum lays down such forward models of required movements in order to make them smooth, coordinated and skilful. First, forward models provide a prediction of the sensory consequences of a movement. So comparison with feedback from the appropriate sense organs indicates whether a movement went off as expected. Unlike an inverse filter therefore, even in the early stages of adaptation a forward model will always provide some sort of signal which can be used to control movement, even though it may still be inaccurate. The negative feedback pathway providing reafference from the moving limb signals how the movement actually went off. This can be compared with the delayed output of the model (Fig. 16), and corrections computed. These are used not only to correct the current movement but also to update, and adapt, the internal model for the new conditions.

Secondly, forward models allow you to imagine and rehearse movements without actually making them. It is probable that such purely mental rehearsal can actually improve physical skill. Recent positron emission tomography (PET) measurements of regional cerebral blood flow have shown that the cerebellum is indeed activated under these conditions, and it would be interesting to correlate this with the acquisition of a new skill. A third advantage of this hypothesis that the cerebellum lays down forward models for controlling movements gives rise to clear predictions of the kinds of signals that we would expect it to generate, and these are being energetically pursued in several laboratories.

Conclusion

The cerebellum is the brain's 'autopilot'. Damage to it leads to loss of automatic, properly calibrated and coordinated, skilled movements, rather than paralysis.

The cerebellum is a 'metasystem'. It receives extensive connections from all the sensory and motor systems. It projects back to the motor cortical areas, red nucleus, vestibular and reticular descending pathways. However, it forms a side loop; it is not on the most direct pathway between any of these sensory or motor structures.

The cerebellum has a regularly repeating matrix-like structure which suggests that despite their different connections all its parts perform a common information processing function.

The interaction of climbing and parallel fibre activity probably regulates the strength of the input from different sources to each Purkinje cell to calibrate movement programmes.

The cerebellum appears to be a sophisticated 'comparator' mediating the sensory calibration of feedforward control systems. By comparing intended movements with those that actually occur it can build up a dossier of internal representations of the dynamic characteristics of the voluntary and reflex motor systems, which are then used to predict the outcome of movements, and hence to perfect their skilled performance.

References

1. Ungerleider, L.G. and Haxby, J. (1992) What and where in the human brain. Curr. Opin. Neurobiol. **4**, 151–159
2. Andersen, R.A. (1987) Inferior parietal lobule function in spatial perception and visuomotor integration. in: Handbook of Physiology, vol. 5, part 2, (Plum, F. and Mountcastle, V.B., eds.), pp. 483–518, Am. Physiol. Soc., Rockville, MD
3. Zipser, D. and Andersen, R.A. (1988) A back-propagation programmed network that simulates response properties of a subset of posterior parietal neurons. Nature (London) **331**, 679–684
4. Stein, J.F. (1992) The representation of egocentric space in the posterior parietal cortex. Behav. Brain Sci. **15**, 691–700
5. Stein, J.F. (1991) Vision and Visual Dyslexia, Macmillan, London
6. Stein, J.F. and Glickstein, M. (1992) The role of the cerebellum in the visual guidance of movement. Physiol. Rev. **72**, 967–1018
7. Ito, M. (1989) Long-term depression. Annu. Rev. Neurosci. **12**, 85–102
8. Allen, G.I. and Tsukahara, M. (1974) Cerebrocerebellar communication systems. Physiol. Rev. **54**, 957–1006
9. Holmes, G. (1939) The cerebellum of man. Brain **62**, 1–30
10. Miall, R.C., Weir, D.J., Wolpert, D.M. and Stein, J.F. (1993) Is the cerebellum a Smith Predictor? J. Motor Behav. **25**, 203–216

4

Compensatory reflex mechanisms following limb displacements

Volker Dietz

Swiss Paraplegic Centre, University Hospital Balgrist, Forchstr. 340, CH-8008 Zürich, Switzerland

Introduction

During the performance of functional movements it is essential that rapid, automatic compensation is made for unexpected external disturbances in order to achieve the desired movement trajectory. This is especially so during highly skilled movements which require an optimal motor performance. Although the neuronal mechanisms underlying these compensatory reactions have been studied for more than 30 years some aspects are still a matter of controversy.

A common approach to the study of these compensatory reactions is to stretch a voluntarily activated muscle. Most of these investigations have been performed on intrinsic hand or forearm muscles. Fig. 1(a) shows the segmented electromyographic (EMG) response that appears in the stretched muscle. The different peaks are labelled M1 to M3 (after [1]) and are followed by a voluntary reaction (labelled 'vol'). Most studies have concentrated on the neuronal basis of the long-latency, or polysynaptic, EMG component 'M2' of the compensatory reaction. The M1 EMG response is generally believed to be mediated by the fast-conducting group-I fibres on a segmental spinal level, as indicated diagrammatically in Fig. 1(b). The M3 EMG response is inconsistent and is therefore neglected in most of the investigations. One major question concerns the pathway of the compensatory M2 response. Is this EMG response also mediated by group-I afferents but on a transcortical pathway, resulting in the longer delay of 25–30 ms compared with the M1 response?

The behaviour of the long-latency response M2 is not only of interest for neurophysiologists but also for clinical neurologists because this EMG response is altered in patients with motor disorders; for example, in patients with spastic paresis or in Parkinson's disease (see [1]). Fig. 2 compares the EMG responses obtained in a patient with Parkinson's disease and those of a normal subject. In the normal subject there was no significant response when the non-activated muscle was stretched. Only following stretch of the activated muscle was there a segmented (M1–M3) EMG response. In the patient with Parkinson's disease two major differences were seen [1]. First, there was no difference in the appearance of the EMG response between the passive and active muscle and secondly, the size of the M2 response was increased. These differences correspond with the clinical signs of poorly modulated motor performance and an increased, more rigid muscle tone.

Beside muscle stretch there are various other methodological approaches that can be used to activate these reflex mechanisms and to study the behaviour of the long-latency EMG response [2]. These include using electrical stimulation of mixed and sensory fibres or platform perturbations and have led to somewhat divergent observations and thus to confusing nomenclature. The present section will deal with the extent to which the behaviour of the long-latency EMG response depends upon (i) the site of the recordings, i.e. whether they were made on the upper or lower limb, or on distal or proximal muscle; and (ii) the influence of the motor task on the response pattern, i.e. to what extent does this determine (a) the selection of afferent fibres for the generation of the EMG response, (b) the reflex pathway for these responses (i.e. spinal or transcortical) and, (c) the processing of the afferent input by the actual motor task.

Afferent fibres

For hand and forearm muscles there is a general agreement that the long-latency, or polysynap-

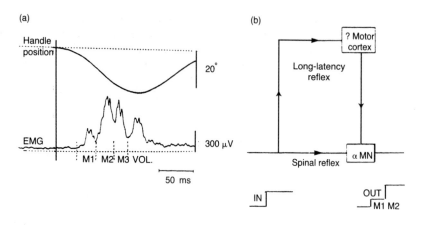

(a) Handle position

20°

EMG

300 μV

M1 M2 M3 VOL.

50 ms

(b)

? Motor cortex

Long-latency reflex

α MN

Spinal reflex

IN

OUT M1 M2

Fig. 1. Stretch-reflex responses

(a) The complex segmented EMG response seen on stretching a human muscle during its voluntary contraction. Top: stimulus applied to the wrist extensor muscles. Bottom: EMG response with separable M1–M3 components preceding any voluntary response. EMG is rectified and averaged, and zero, is indicated by a dashed line. (b) A schematic diagram illustrating how the delay of the M2 response might arise (Reproduced with permission from [8]).

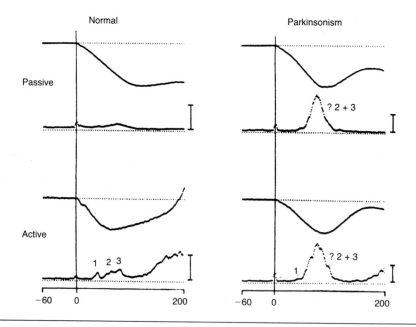

Normal

Parkinsonism

Passive

? 2 + 3

Active

1 2 3

? 2 + 3

1

−60   0   200

−60   0   200

Fig. 2. Stretch reflex responses in normal subject and patient with Parkinson's disease

EMG responses to sudden wrist displacements in a normal subject and a patient with Parkinson's disease. For each subject the passive task is above and the active task below. The top trace of each pair shows the average handle position (flexion downward) and the bottom trace is the averaged rectified EMG response (calibration in mV) from the wrist extensors. The torque motor was turned on at time 0 (abscissa, calibration in ms). (Reproduced with permission from [1]).

tic, EMG responses are mediated by the fast-conducting group-Ia fibres. This suggestion is supported by several observations. One of the most convincing is shown in Fig. 3. The onset latencies of the M1 and M2 responses are plotted against the height of the subject. It becomes obvious from this figure that the slope for the M2 responses parallels that of the M1 responses. This indicates that the M2 responses are mediated by the same fibres as the M1 responses, i.e. by group-I afferent fibres. If the M2 responses were mediated, for example, by slower-conducting group-II fibres, proportionally longer latencies would be expected with increasing height, i.e. the slope of the M2 response regression line would be expected to be steeper [3].

These observations hold for the forearm muscles. But when a similar methodological approach is applied to the lower leg, with stretching of the activated leg extensor muscles by a torque motor, different results are seen [4]. Fig. 4 shows the soleus EMG responses following stretch of the activated soleus muscle. The early response M1 was not followed by a corresponding M2 response. An activation of the gastrocnemius occurred only after more than 140 ms.

A long-latency EMG response with a latency (65–75 ms) corresponding to that seen in the arm muscles appeared in the lower leg muscles when the stretch was applied during functional movements, i.e. during perturbations of stance or gait [5]. Fig. 5 shows the gastrocnemius EMG responses following three different modes of stretch. In Fig. 5(a) the passive muscle was stretched resulting only in the appearance of an early EMG response. When the same subject was standing on a treadmill and a backward displacement of the support-surface was applied, stretching the gastrocnemius (Fig. 5b), the small early response was followed by a strong gastrocnemius activation which appeared with a latency of about 70 ms. When the same perturbation was induced at the

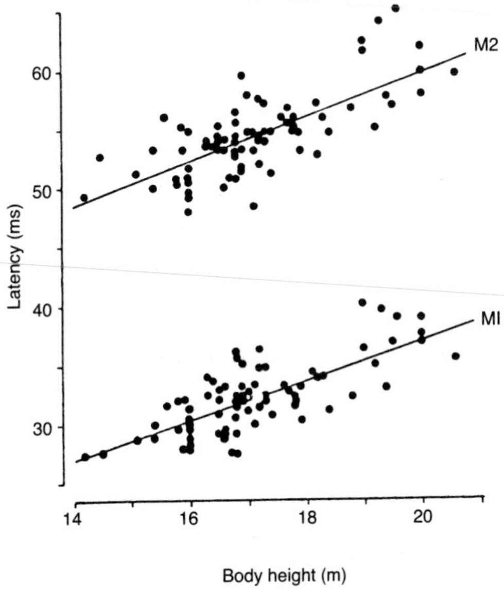

Fig. 3. Response latencies and body height

Dependence of latency of the M1 and M2 responses in the first dorsal interosseus muscle on body height of 77 subjects. Latencies were measured between onset of small transient stretch (1°) and onset of reflex response. Linear regression lines yielded the following parameters: slope (b) and ordinate intercept (a) given with 95% confidence limits. M1: r = 0.70 (P<0.001), b = 16.6ms/m, a = 21.7ms; M2: r = 0.72 (P<0.001), b = 19ms/m, a = 3.8ms. (Reproduced with permission from [3]).

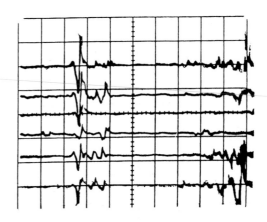

Fig. 4. Stretch reflex responses in soleus muscle

Successive raw EMG responses recorded in the soleus muscle evoked by different levels of sudden forced dorsiflexion of the foot. Two separate responses may be seen when the subject is instructed to resist as quickly as possible, one starting at 50ms and the other after 140ms. Grid divisions are 1mV and 20ms. Oscilloscope sweep triggered at the torque onset. (Reproduced with permission from [4]).

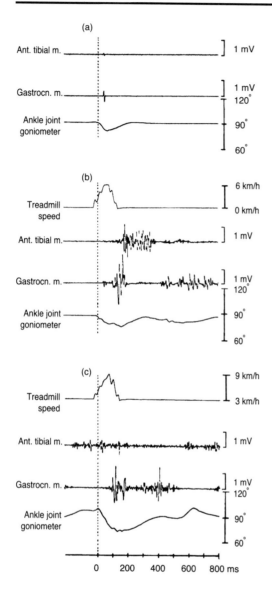

Fig. 5. Gastrocnemius EMG responses to stretch in three different tasks

Raw recordings of gastrocnemius muscle EMG responses following different types of displacements (foot dorsiflexion) in the same subject together with ankle joint movements. (a) Passive foot dorsiflexion of the relaxed leg. (b) Positive acceleration impulse of the treadmill applied during standing and (c) during gait (3km/h). (Reproduced with permission from [5]).

beginning of stance phase of gait (Fig. 5c) the early response was absent and only a long-latency EMG response appeared in the leg extensor muscles.

According to investigations exploiting the H-reflex technique [6], the absence of the early response is probably due to an increased presynaptic inhibition of the group-Ia afferents which is stronger during gait than during stance (cf. [6]). These observations make it unlikely that the long-latency EMG response in the gastrocnemius during the functional movement is mediated by group-Ia afferents. Further support comes from experiments in which the group-I afferents were blocked while the efferent motor axons to the leg muscles could still conduct impulses [7]. Under these conditions the compensatory long-latency EMG response was preserved. As shown in Fig. 6, the EMG response following ischaemic blocking of group-I afferents was quite similar to the response obtained without blocking during self-induced or randomly induced perturbations. This suggests that this response is mediated by fibres which are more resistant to ischaemia, i.e. by fibres of smaller diameter and slower conduction velocity (group-II or -III afferents).

▶ For hand and forearm muscles the long-latency EMG responses are mediated by group-Ia afferent fibres.
▶ For the leg extensor muscles (e.g. gastrocnemius) the compensatory long-latency EMG response following a perturbation of stance and gait is mediated by fibres other than group Ia afferents (most probably by group-II and/or -III afferents).

Reflex pathways

There are several observations which indicate that in hand and forearm muscles the M2 response is mediated via a transcortical pathway (for review see [8]). Two observations supporting this view arise from patients with motor disorders. The first comes from subjects who display mirror movements, i.e. voluntary movements of one hand are accompanied by involuntary movements of the contralateral side. Fig. 7 shows that stretching the activated first dorsal interosseous muscle of one side was followed by long-latency EMG responses

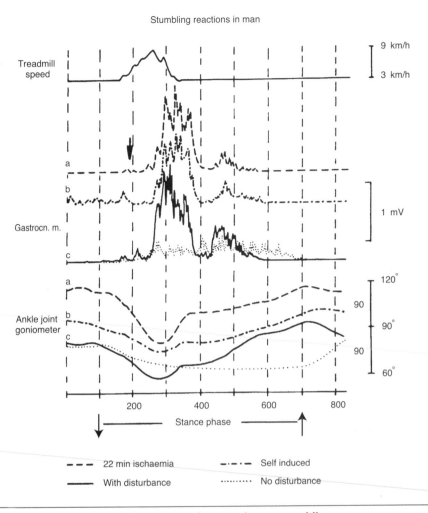

Fig. 6. Behaviour of the corrective reaction to stumbling

Rectified and averaged (n = 16) gastrocnemius EMG and ankle joint movements following acceleration of the treadmill 80 ms after heel contact in three different conditions: a, after 22 min of ischaemia; b, acceleration initiated by the volunteer; c, acceleration unexpectedly induced. The dotted line represents the undisturbed walking pattern. The arrow indicates the time of onset of the effective change in belt speed. The arrows below the Figure indicate touch-down and lift-up of the respective foot. (Reproduced with permission from [7]).

which appeared with about the same latency on both sides. The M1 response was seen only on the stretched side. This suggests that the M2 response in these subjects is mediated on a transcortical pathway and appears on both sides, due perhaps to an abnormal branching of the efferent axons originating from supraspinal motor centres (see [8]). This is shown schematically in Fig. 7(b).

Further support for this view comes from patients with Huntington's Chorea, an inherited motor disorder manifest as degeneration of supraspinal motor centres. Clinically, the presence of continuous generalized involuntary movements is one of the prominent symptoms of this disease. Fig. 8(a) shows that on stretching of the first dorsal interosseous of a Huntington's patient only an M1 response was

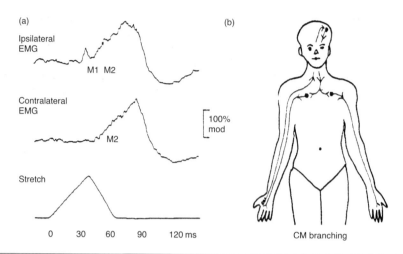

Fig. 7. Stretch reflex responses in distal arm muscle
(a) The bilateral occurrence of the long-latency EMG response of the first dorsal interosseus in a patient with mirror movements. Note that the stretched muscle gave a small M1 response. (b) A possible neuronal circuit that may underlie the results shown in (a). The descending corticomotoneuronal fibres of the pyramidal tract show abnormal branching to supply corresponding motoneurons on both sides of the spinal cord. (Reproduced with permission from [8]).

seen. The M2 response was absent. This was interpreted as being due to an interruption of the transcortical pathway [9]. However, when more proximal muscles (biceps brachii) were stretched in the same patient the M2 response appeared in the stretched muscle with a similar latency and amplitude as in normal subjects (Fig. 8b). The latter observation indicates that the long-latency EMG response in more proximal arm muscles is mediated by a separate pathway, for example, a spinal pathway [10].

For the lower leg muscles, a spinal pathway of the long-latency EMG response should be present as the onset latency of 65–75 ms is too short for a supraspinal pathway [7], taking into account that this response is mediated by fibres which are slower-conducting than group-Ia fibres (see above).

> ▶ In hand and forearm muscles the long-latency (M2) response is mediated via a transcortical pathway.
> ▶ For the lower leg muscles, a spinal pathway of the long-latency EMG response should be present.

Selection and processing of afferent input

To investigate the influence of the actual motor task on the behaviour of the long-latency EMG response (see [11]), subjects were asked to perform sinusoidal isometric contractions of biceps and triceps brachii muscles (Fig. 9). In one condition, the subjects were asked to hold the elbow joint angle at a constant angle of 90 ° while a sinusoidal torque was applied to the flexor and extensor muscles. In the other condition, the elbow joint angle was held constant by the motor and the subject was asked to exert a sinusoidally changing torque using the flexors and extensors. During their main activity phase, the flexor or extensor muscles were stretched at different velocities (indicated by the arrows in Fig. 9).

The EMG responses following stretch of the flexors are displayed in Fig. 9. The EMG responses in the brachioradialis muscle were different depending upon whether elbow position (Fig. 9a) or torque (Fig. 9b) was controlled by the subject. During subject's control of elbow position a monosynaptic EMG response was followed by a long-latency EMG response. The rate of rise of the latter response was dependent upon the stretch velocity. The increase of this EMG response always ended at about the same time regardless of stretch velocity. In contrast, the EMG responses obtained during subjects' control of torque consisted of a plateau, the amplitude of which was dependent

on the stretch velocity. The duration of the plateau corresponded to the duration of stretch. Overall, the EMG responses during control of position were larger than those during control of torque. In addition, during control of position, there was a closer correlation of the EMG responses with the acceleration signal while during the control of torque the closest correla-

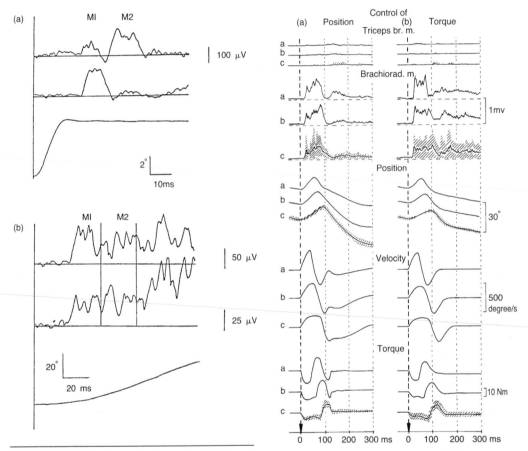

Fig. 8. Stretch reflex responses in distal and proximal arm muscles

(a) Rectified and averaged (n=128) EMG records obtained following stretch (5° at a rate of 400°/s) of the first dorsal interosseus of a normal subject (upper trace) and a patient with Huntington's Chorea (middle trace). (Reproduced with permission from [9]). (b) Rectified and averaged (n=10) EMG record obtained following stretch (30° at a rate of 300°/s) of the biceps brachii of a normal subject (upper trace) and a patient with Huntington's Chorea (middle trace). The vertical lines indicate the M2 interval (45–85ms). The lower traces in (a) and (b) show the imposed displacement (from [10]).

Fig. 9. Task-dependent modulation of stretch reflex response in proximal arm muscle

Group averages (±S.D. for impulse c, shaded area) of the rectified and averaged (n=10 trials) arm muscle EMG responses, together with position, velocity and torque signals, following various extending displacements induced during sinusoidal isometric muscle contractions while subjects controlled the elbow position (a) or elbow torque (b) for 15 subjects. Displacement amplitude was fixed at 12° and velocity at a, 300; b, 200; and c, 150°/s (impulses a–c). Arrows indicate onset of displacement. (Reproduced with permission from [11]).

tion was obtained with the velocity signal [11]. It is suggested that the difference in the EMG responses seen in the two motor tasks is due to selection of afferent input from, for example, stretch or load receptors coupled with an appropriate processing of the afferent input.

A similar influence of the actual motor task was also seen during perturbations of stance. A common approach used to study the compensatory reactions following stance perturbation is to induce platform rotations (e.g. feet dorsiflexions) or platform translations (e.g. backward-going feet translations). The compensatory reactions following these perturbations of stance were quite different (see Fig. 10) although the stretch applied to activated leg extensor muscles was about the same between

the two conditions [12]. During feet dorsiflexing platform rotations (Fig. 10a), a small early gastrocnemius response was followed by tibialis anterior activation. This pattern of tibialis anterior muscle activation resulted in compensation for the backward sway of the body and thus balance was maintained. During backward translations (Fig. 10b), the support surface was displaced under the body's centre of mass. A strong, functionally essential, gastrocnemius activity appeared with a latency of about 70–80 ms. The latter EMG response is needed to hold the body's centre of mass over the feet. It has been suggested by Nashner [13] that the difference in the compensatory reactions between rotational and translational perturbations is due to a reflex adaptation within four to

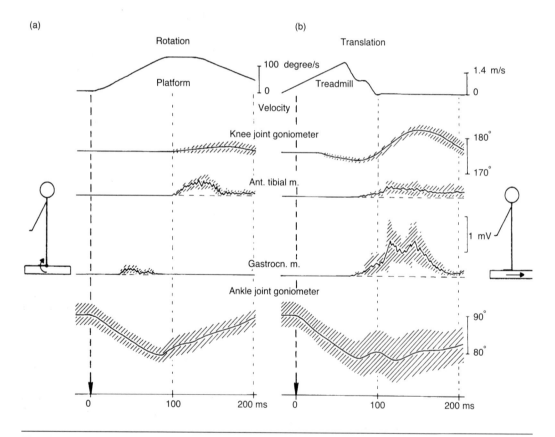

Fig. 10. Task-dependent modulation of stretch reflex responses in lower leg muscles
Mean (± S.D., shaded area) of rectified and averaged (n = 30) leg muscle EMG responses together with knee and ankle joint movements, of seven subjects following a dorsiflexing rotations of the platform (a) and a backward translation of the treadmill (b). (Reproduced with permission from [12]).

five trials after the change. A gastrocnemius activation becomes established during backward translations, but following dorsiflexing platform rotation this activity disappears with successive trials. Recent experiments failed to support this concept of adaptation (for review see [2]). Instead, it was proposed that the qualitatively appropriate pattern is already present from the first trial even when the two conditions are applied randomly. It was claimed that an additional afferent input is necessary for the generation of the appropriate response.

To get further information about this additional afferent input, two different modes of dorsiflexing platform rotations were applied. One involved rotations about the ankle joint while the other involved inducing translational (backward) movements. These displacements were applied while the body was in a supine position in order to exclude vestibular influence [14]. When pure rotational impulses were applied only small early EMG responses appeared in the gastrocnemius muscle (Fig. 11a) similar to those seen during vertical body posture (see Fig. 10a). However, following displacements with a translational component, a strong long-latency EMG response appeared in the leg extensor muscles (Fig. 11b). The size of the long-latency EMG response in the gastrocnemius depended upon the force with which the body was pressed at the shoulders against the platform. This dependency of the EMG response on the loading of the body indicates that the presence and strength of the long-latency EMG response depends on the additional torque exerted on the extensor muscles by the displacement according to the formula: $T = l \times r$ (T = torque; l = load; r = translation distance).

These findings suggest that afferent input from load receptors in leg extensor muscles contribute to the functionally essential long-latency responses in the leg extensor muscles. This agrees with the findings of Pearson and Collins [15] which indicated that extensor load receptors activate the leg extensor muscles and interact with spinal generators responsible for locomotion. These receptors most probably correspond with the Golgi tendon organs with a presumed impulse transmission by group-Ib afferents.

▶ Afferent input from load receptors contribute to the functionally essential long-latency EMG responses in the leg extensor muscles during gait.
▶ A selection and processing of afferent input takes place at a spinal level that is further subject to control by supraspinal centres. This selection depends on the actual motor task.

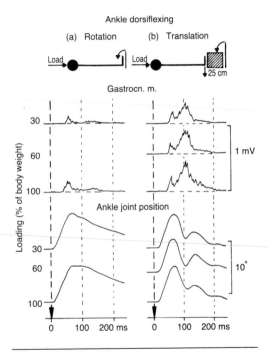

Fig. 11. Influence of contact force on stretch reflex responses in lower leg muscle
Mean of rectified and averaged (n=10) leg muscle EMG responses together with the ankle joint position of 10 subjects following a dorsiflexing rotation of the platform co-linear with the ankle joint (a), and with the ankle joints 25cm above the rotational axis (b). The perturbations were applied with the body in a supine position. The subjects were pressed at the shoulders against the platform by 30, 60 and 100% of their body weight. (Reproduced with permission from [14]).

Conclusions

▶ There are several observations which suggest that the long-latency EMG response (M2) in hand and forearm muscles is mediated by group-I afferents. However, the compensatory long-latency EMG response in the leg extensor muscles following stretch, induced during functional movements, is more likely to be mediated by fibres other than group-Ia afferents.

▶ We have to be aware that afferent input from stretch receptors (mediated by group-Ia or group-II fibres) is not the sole contributor to functionally essential EMG responses. There is increasing evidence that load receptors within the extensor muscles (probably Golgi tendon organs) also contribute to the generation of the long-latency EMG responses. The selection and processing of the respective afferent inputs probably takes place at a spinal level that is further subject to control by supraspinal centres.

▶ Recent experimental data indicate that different mechanisms underlie the generation of M2 stretch-reflex response in distal and proximal arm muscles. Distal hand muscles are probably mediated via a transcortical pathway, while there are observations which indicate a spinal pathway for proximal arm and lower leg muscles.

This work was supported by the Swiss National Science Foundation (grant no. 31-33567.92).

References

1. Lee, R.G. and Tatton, W.G. (1975) Motor responses to sudden limb displacements in primates with specific CNS lesions and in human patients with motor system disorders. Can. J. Neurol. Sci. 2, 285–293
2. Dietz, V. (1992) Human neuronal control of automatic functional movements: interaction between central programs and afferent input. Physiol. Rev. 72, 33–69
3. Noth, J., Schwarz, M., Podoll, K. and Motamedi, F. (1991) Evidence that low-threshold muscle afferents evoke long-latency stretch reflexes in human hand muscles. J. Neurophysiol. 65, 1089–1097
4. Gottlieb, G.L. and Agarwal, G.C. (1979) Response to sudden torques about ankle in man: myotactic reflex. J. Neurophysiol. 42, 91–106
5. Dietz, V., Quintern, J. and Berger, W. (1984) Corrective reactions to stumbling in man: functional significance of spinal and transcortical reflexes. Neurosci. Lett. 44, 131–135
6. Stein, R.B. and Capaday, C. (1988) The modulation of human reflexes during functional motor tasks. Trends Neurosci. 11, 328–332
7. Berger, W., Dietz, V. and Quintern, J. (1984) Corrective reactions to stumbling in man: neuronal coordination of bilateral leg muscle activity during gait. J. Physiol. (London) 357, 109–125
8. Matthews, P.B.C., Farmer, S.F. and Ingram, D.A. (1990) On the localization of the stretch reflex of intrinsic hand muscles in a patient with mirror movements. J. Physiol. (London) 428, 561–577
9. Noth, J., Podoll, K. and Friedemann, H.H. (1985) Long-loop reflexes in small hand muscles studied in normal subjects and in patients with Huntington's disease. Brain 108, 65–80
10. Thilmann, A.F., Schwarz, M., Töpper, R., Fellows, S.J. and Noth, J. (1991) Different mechanisms underlie the long-latency stretch reflex response of active human muscle at different joints. J. Physiol. (London) 444, 631–643
11. Dietz, V., Trippel, M. and Berger, W. (1991) Reflex activity and muscle tone during elbow movements in patients with spastic paresis. Ann. Neurol. 30, 767–779
12. Dietz, V., Trippel, M., Discher, M. and Horstmann, G.A. (1991) Compensation of human stance perturbations: selection of the appropriate electromyographic pattern. Neurosci. Lett. 126, 71–74
13. Nashner, L.M. (1976) Adapting reflexes controlling the human posture. Exp. Brain Res. 26, 59–72
14. Dietz, V., Gollhofer, A., Kleiber, M. and Trippel, M. (1992) Regulation of bipedal stance: dependency on 'load' receptors. Exp. Brain Res. 89, 229–231
15. Pearson, K.G. and Collins, D.F. (1993) Reversal of the influence of group Ib afferents from plantaris on activity in medial gastrocnemius muscle during locomotor activity. J. Neurophysiol. 70, 1009–1017

5

The control of speech

David H. McFarland*† and James P. Lund‡
*École d'Orthophonie et d'Audiologie et Centre de Recherche en Sciences Neurologique, Faculté de Médecine, Université de Montréal, C.P. 6128, succ. Centre-Ville, Montréal, Québec, Canada H3C 3J7 and ‡Faculty of Dentistry, McGill University, 3640 University Street, Montréal, Québec, Canada H3A 2BZ

Introduction

Speech differs from many other skilled movements (with the exception of sign language), in that the goal is not to move the body or an object but to communicate. During a conversation, we listen and attempt to understand what is being said by the other speaker. We usually formulate at least part of our reply before beginning to speak, and this language is then translated into speech sounds.

It has been estimated that we may produce up to 12 of these sounds per second during normal conversation, and this may require the activity of up to 100 muscles distributed across several motor systems. This makes speech one of the most complex of all skilled human behaviours, and poses a particular problem for those who wish to understand the underlying control mechanisms. Although speech and sound generation are not strictly comparable, many of the substrates for speech are present in other animals that communicate through sound (e.g. birds, dolphins and non-human primates).

In this chapter, we will first describe the different types of speech sounds and the three musculoskeletal systems involved in their production. We will then review the neural control of vocalization in birds and non-human primates, making comparisons to man whenever possible, before finally focusing on the cortical, sub-cortical and peripheral neural components of the human speech control system.

Speech sound generation

Types of speech sounds

The study of speech sound generation has enjoyed a colourful history. Much of what we know about the features of specific speech sounds can be traced back to John Wilkins, Dean of Rippon, and Alexander Melville Bell, Professor of Vocal Physiology and Lecturer on Elocution at University College, London.

In 1668, John Wilkins published an essay on language requested by the Royal Society [1]. It is a marvellous concoction of theology, philosophy and scientific observation that begins with a description of the origins of language in the garden of Eden, the multiplication of tongues in the confusion of Babel, and their dispersion by the families of Noah. Even a detailed diagram of the Ark showing the stabling of its inhabitants was provided. Wilkins, however, was a keen observer, and he clearly recognized the difference between language formation and speech, the motor act. He described how many of the speech sounds are produced (see ref. [1] pages 358–380) and illustrated these events in a detailed woodcut (Fig. 1). As shown in this Figure, speech sounds are generated by coordinated activity in the respiratory, laryngeal and articulatory systems. The term 'articulatory system', as used by speech scientists, refers to the supralaryngeal vocal tract (e.g. pharynx, soft palate, jaws, lips and tongue).

Speech sounds are classified as 'voiced' or 'unvoiced'. The distinction involves the presence (voiced) or absence (unvoiced) of the sound created by the vibration of the vocal folds. Wilkins indicated this voicing by drawing the outline of the epiglottis on the neck of the Figure for the 'b' sound, because he mistakenly believed that voicing arose from vibrations of the epiglottis. All English vowels and some consonants (e.g. 'd') are voiced, while the remaining consonant sounds (e.g. 't') are unvoiced.

Unlike tonal languages, such as Chinese, the different speech sounds of English are not distinguished by their pitch; that is, they are not dependent on the fundamental frequency of vocal fold vibration. Instead, the acoustic cues that distinguish particular voiced sounds, such as vowels, are generated when the vibrating air

† To whom correspondence should be addressed.

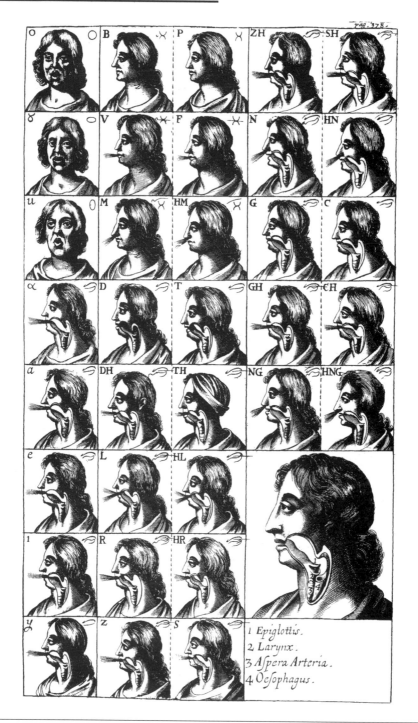

Fig. I. Speech sound generation according to John Wilkins 1668

Woodcut showing the generation of many of the speech sounds. Vowels are illustrated in the far left column. In the upper right-hand corner of each figure are drawn the positions of the lips or the direction of the airflow within the oral cavity. See text for additional details.

column is shaped by the active and passive characteristics of the vocal tract (see Figs. 1 and 4).

To form unvoiced sounds, the vocal tract functions as the sound generator. The lips, teeth and tongue are used to constrict and/or close-off and release the airflow. For example, the sound 's' (bottom right of Wilkins' Figure) or 'sh' (upper right) is produced when the airstream is directed against the incisal edge of the upper or lower teeth to create turbulence. The passage of the airstream over the tip of the tongue is shown schematically in the upper right corners of the drawings for the 's' and 'sh' sounds in the Wilkins' Figure. For other sounds (referred to as 'stops'), the blocking of flow is complete and followed by a rapid release. An example of this type of sound is the 'p' in which intra-oral air pressure builds up behind the lips and is then released. The curved lines in the upper right corner of the drawing of the 'p' sound in the Wilkins' Figure indicates bilabial closure. The 'b' sound is produced similarly, except that there is voicing immediately after the first sound burst.

The nasal cavity has special resonant properties which characterize sounds such as 'n' and 'm', and these sounds are produced with the nasopharynx coupled to the rest of the vocal tract. Note the airflow through the nose for these nasalized sounds in Wilkins' drawings.

Systems involved in speech sound generation

In 1867 Alexander Melville Bell published 'Visible Speech' which was an alphabetical code of the positions and movements that speech articulators made to generate each sound [2]. The code was written as a universal language and as a visible speech aid for the deaf. His son Alexander Graham Bell (the inventor of the telephone), continued the family interest in the mechanics of speech production and deaf education. Both his mother and wife were deaf.

Alexander Melville Bell was a careful observer of the speech production process and the systems involved in speech sound generation. He noted: "The lungs constitute the bellows of the speaking machine; the larynx, the pharynx, the soft palate, the nose and the mouth, modify the breath into the elementary sounds of speech" ([2] p. 11). We will elaborate on these speech functions in the following sections.

The respiratory system

As Bell proposed, the role of the respiratory system in speech is to create pressure in the upper airway [3]. During conversation, the pressure beneath the closed vocal folds (subglottal pressure) is maintained within a relatively narrow range, although we can modulate this up and down to control prosodic elements, such as loudness. The maintenance of a constant subglottal pressure involves a complex interaction between the forces generated by the passive mechanical properties of the lungs and thorax, and those generated by the active contraction of respiratory muscles. This interaction is most easily illustrated using the example of an opera singer who has to sustain a sound at a relatively constant loudness for a long time. To do this, the singer inspires to very high lung volumes, initiates the sound, and continues to very low volumes. At high lung volumes, however, subglottal pressures generated solely by the passive relaxation characteristics of the lungs and thorax exceed those needed for the task. If the relaxation of the chest at these high volumes was not opposed by restraining forces, the sound would be loud and very short, because the singer would soon run out of breath. To maintain the utterance, inspiratory muscles must contract to counterbalance the passive recoil of the tissues. As the utterance continues, volume decreases and the passive pressure falls, so the restraining action of inspiratory muscles must decrease continuously and proportionately. At a certain volume, the relaxed chest and lungs actually generate negative or inspiratory pressure, and expiratory muscles must now contract to maintain phonation. We have drawn Fig. 2 to depict these interactions. As shown, it seems likely that there must be at least some overlap in the activity of inspiratory and expiratory muscles during a sustained utterance, thereby creating a stiffer system which would make the control of expiratory flow easier. Co-contraction of agonist and antagonist muscles is a common feature of many types of movements, such as slow movements of the arm and hand. There is kinematic evidence that abdominal muscles and the diaphragm are co-activated when inspiration occurs during normal conversation. This probably allows the diaphragmatic muscle fibres to work within the optimal portion of their length-tension curve. Consequently, the diaphragm can draw in air more efficiently and rapidly, which probably

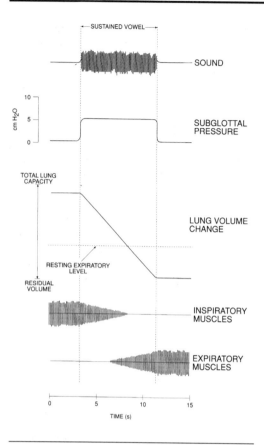

Fig. 2. Diagram showing the production of a sustained vowel initiated at high lung volumes and continued to low lung volumes

When the lungs are full, subglottal pressure generated solely by the passive relaxation characteristics of the lungs and thorax exceed that needed for the task, so inspiratory muscles must contract as a counterbalance. At low volumes, subglottal pressure is maintained by contraction of expiratory muscles.

helps to shorten inspiratory pauses during speech.

We do not take very large breaths during normal speech (unlike singing), and inspirations typically terminate just above the end-inspiratory level of quiet breathing, although we do tend to increase inspiratory volume when speaking loudly. Inspiration typically occurs at phrase and sentence boundaries to minimize interruptions to the flow of conversation.

Because speech is produced during expiration, this phase is longer and associated with lower flow rates than during quiet breathing.

Depending upon linguistic demands, contraction of expiratory muscles may be used to force the system to lung volumes well below the end-expiratory level of quiet breathing.

The laryngeal system

The larynx has two primary biological functions. First, it prevents foreign objects from entering the airway, and secondly, it traps air in the filled lungs to stabilize the torso for activities such as lifting heavy objects and childbirth. Superimposed on these primitive functions is the use of the vocal folds in the generation of speech sounds. Much effort has been expended in describing and modelling the vocal folds and the factors that change their vibratory characteristics. For our purposes, we will use a simplified description of the process (Fig. 3). First of all, it is important to note that vocal fold vibration is not caused by cyclical activity in laryngeal muscles. Instead, intrinsic and extrinsic laryngeal muscles contract tonically to bring the vocal folds to their closed position. Vibration results from the interaction of aerodynamic forces and the elastic characteristics of vocal fold tissues [4].

To produce voiced sounds, the vocal folds are closed and subglottal pressure is allowed to build up until it overcomes the resistance of the closed folds, releasing a burst of compressed air into the supraglottal space (Fig. 3) [5]. Bernoulli forces, coupled with the elastic recoil of the stretched tissue, return the folds to their closed position. The cycle repeats itself when subglottal pressure again overcomes the forces that adduct the vocal folds. Driven by these puffs, the air above the larynx vibrates. The rate at which the vocal folds open and close determines the fundamental frequency (F_O) of vibration, and consequently of the voice. The perceptual correlate of F_O is pitch. The vocal folds not only open and close, they vibrate in a complex manner. This gives rise to a sound spectrum (Fig. 4) that contains the F_O and higher-order harmonics with significant energy up to about 4500 Hz.

The thyroid cartilage is bigger in males than in females (this is why the 'Adam's apple' is more prominent in males), in order to support longer and more massive vocal folds. Long, heavy vocal folds vibrate more slowly than short, light ones, and this explains why F_O is much lower in most adult males than in females (approximately 130 Hz versus 260 Hz).

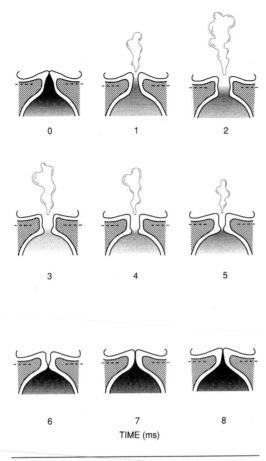

0 1 2

3 4 5

6 7 8

TIME (ms)

Fig. 3. Diagram showing a single cycle of vocal fold vibration

Pressure increases until it overcomes the resistance of the closed vocal folds, releasing a burst of compressed air into the vocal tract (modified from [17] and [5]). Bernoulli forces, coupled with the elastic recoil of the stretched tissue, return the folds to their closed position, and the cycle repeats itself.

It is the rapid changes in the length and thickness of the vocal folds of boys during puberty that causes the voice to 'break'.

Changing F_O is important for song and for effective communication during conversational speech. A rising F_O at the end of a sentence signifies a question, and we can usually tell the state of someone's mood from the F_O of the voice. Changes in F_O result mainly from changes in the length/tension characteristics of the vibrating folds. Although the exact mechanisms by which this is achieved are not completely understood, it seems likely that the cricothyroid, an extrinsic laryngeal muscle, acts to lengthen the vocal folds, while the contraction of the thyroarytenoid muscles (which make up the main mass of the vibrating folds) increases tension. Increasing subglottal pressure may also influence F_O, but this may not be as significant as laryngeal adjustments.

The intensity of speech, which is perceived as loudness, is determined primarily by changes in subglottal pressure. To increase vocal intensity, the vocal folds are more tightly closed, and greater respiratory drive is generated to overcome the added resistance. The proportion of time that the vocal folds are open during a given vibratory cycle decreases as intensity increases, and the amplitude of vibration of the vocal folds increases. This results in an increase in the number of harmonics and in the energy that they carry. This 'voicing spectrum' is then modified by the supraglottal vocal tract and articulatory structures to produce specific sounds (Fig. 4).

The articulatory system

The sounds created by vocal fold vibration (voiced sounds) are given meaning by changing the configuration of the vocal tract, which acts as a filter with modifiable resonant modes (Fig. 4). Those frequencies at or near these resonant modes (called formant frequencies) pass most effectively, while others are attenuated. Consequently, the frequency spectrum of the glottal sound source is modified as it passes through the filter. The filter characteristics of the upper vocal tract depend on its shape, which in turn, is controlled by muscular action.

Vowels are formed with the vocal tract relatively open and are differentiated by their distinct spectral characteristics. Specifically, the first three formants appear to distinguish the different vowels. Consonants are more complex sounds that require rapid movements of one or more of the speech articulators (e.g. jaws, lips and tongue) to close-off and/or constrict the vocal tract. These movements create transient and/or turbulent sounds that distinguish the various consonants.

Dynamics

Vocal tract configuration changes as the articulators move from the production of one speech sound to the next, and the articulatory features of different sounds may overlap in time. That is, articulators may be moving to produce a future

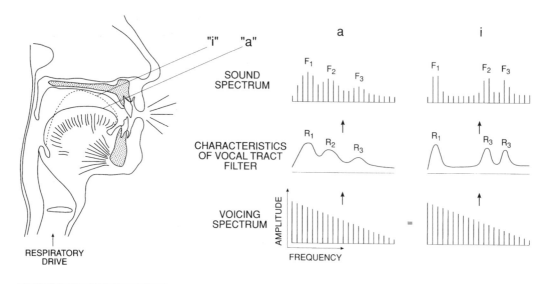

Fig. 4. Filter characteristics of the upper vocal tract

Vowels are distinguished because of changes that occur in the spectrum of the voicing source as it passes through the vocal tract. The vocal tract is a filter with modifiable resonant modes (R). Changes in the configuration of the vocal tract alter the resonant modes, and those frequencies at or near R, called formant frequencies (F), pass most effectively. In general, each vowel is associated with particular vocal tract configurations. We illustrate how the same voicing spectrum is transformed into the sounds 'i' and 'a' by changing vocal tract shape.

sound while the current one is still being generated. This overlap of gestures, which is termed 'co-articulation', has been seen in other complex movement sequences, such as typing. Co-articulation is indicative of the flexibility and context-dependency of speech articulation, and of the fact that there are a number of articulatory movements that can give rise to a given sound. To explain this, most theories of speech motor control incorporate in some fashion the notion of 'motor equivalence', which is the principle that many activation patterns or movement trajectories can be used to achieve a given goal. A simple illustration of this principle is throwing a ball; we can do it overhand, underhand, or sidearm and still get it to the target. Any theory of speech motor control must take this into account, as well as the large body of evidence that the system can compensate for a variety of perturbations of the oral environment. A striking example of this is that intelligi-

ble speech can be produced after surgical removal of large portions of the tongue. Other less severe disruptions to the articulatory system also require compensatory behaviours (see peripheral neural mechanisms below).

A question which has occupied the attention of many speech motor control theorists is: What, if any, are the critical features of speech articulation? Some authors argue that the regulated variables are the spatial positions of the articulatory structures, while others suggest that the location and degree of constriction within the vocal tract are controlled. A variant of this is that the overall shape (or length) of the vocal tract is the critical variable. More recently, other scientists have suggested that speech articulation arises from cooperative relationships among muscle synergies. The adaptive nature of articulatory gestures is seen as a natural consequence of the dynamic linkages between the components of the vocal tract.

► Speech is a rapid and dynamic process which demands the simultaneous control of temporally overlapping movements in the respiratory, laryngeal and articulatory systems.

► The respiratory system generates pressure in the upper airway, the laryngeal system functions as a sound source for voiced sounds, and the articulatory system modifies the configuration of the vocal tract to produce specific sounds.

Neural control of animal vocalization

Much of the progress in identifying neural structures potentially involved in speech motor control has been made by studying the neural control of animal vocalization. Even primitive vertebrates vocalize, and brain stem mechanisms that control this behaviour appear to persist in higher species. For example, electrical stimulation of the periaqueductal gray (PAG) elicits sound in mammals, birds, reptiles, amphibians and even fish, and infarcts or lesions in PAG can cause mutism in a variety of species including man. As we review the control of vocalization in birds and non-human primates in the following sections, we will try to emphasize features that are of particular interest to human speech.

Avian vocalization

Of all animal species, the neural control of vocalization has been most extensively studied in birds. Vocal production differs considerably in complexity across avian species and this seems to reflect the level of development of the neural control mechanisms [6]. Many species, such as the domestic hen, have a very limited vocal repertoire that is mainly controlled by the brain stem. This is in stark contrast to oscine songbirds, such as canaries, sparrows and finches, which possess rich and diversified song patterns that are used for intra-species communication [7]. The more complex song patterns typically belong to the males of these species.

Several areas of the brain of oscine species are involved in the patterning and transmission of motor commands to the muscles of the sound-generating apparatus, the syrinx. These

nuclei are interconnected to form a vocal control system that is hierarchically organized (Fig. 5). There also appears to be a left-sided lateralization of song control function. Auditory input to the system comes from ascending auditory pathways that supply the high vocal centre (HVC), a large neostriatal nucleus that participates in both the learning and production of song. Although the HVC is crucial for song production, the initiation command probably arises in the thalamus (Uva) or from even lower centres. The HVC projects to another forebrain nucleus, the robust nucleus of the archistriatum (RA) which, in turn, projects to the motoneurons that innervate the muscles of the syrinx in a specific part of the hypoglossal nucleus

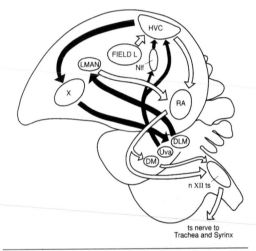

Fig. 5. Neural control of vocalization in song birds

Interrelationships between the different brain structures involved in both the learning and production of song bird vocalization (redrawn from [7]). The HVC–RA–XIIts pathway appears to be of most importance for the production of song, while the recursive loop (HVC–X–DLM–LMAN–RA) is thought to participate in the learning of new songs. Abbreviations used: HVC, high vocal centre; FIELD L, auditory projection of caudal neostriatum; X, area X of lobus parolfactorius; DLM, medial portion of the dorsolateral thalamic nucleus; DM, pars dorsalis medialis of the nucleus intercollicularis; LMAN, lateral magnocellular nucleus of the anterior neostriatum; Nlf, interface nucleus; RA, robust nucleus of the archistriatum; nXIIts, pars tracheosyringealis of the hypoglossal nucleus; ts nerve, tracheosyringealis nerve; Uva, nucleus uvaeformis.

(XIIts). A sub-system, termed the recursive loop, appears to be important for the learning of new song patterns. This pathway also leads from HVC to RA but it passes through several relays in the neostriatum and thalamus (Fig. 5). Lesions of these intermediate nuclei disrupt the learning of new songs.

Many birds appear to learn song in a manner similar to human infants, that is, by imitating auditory models. When song birds are raised in acoustic isolation they develop abnormal patterns called isolate songs. Early deafening in canaries and other species has catastrophic effects on song development, because it limits access to external models. Deafening of adult zebra finches results in a gradual deterioration of song production, presumably because this prevents the monitoring and correction of the bird's own inherited vocal productions.

Oscine species progress through three major stages of song development: subsong, plastic song and stable or adult song. During subsong, the calls are low in intensity and highly variable, as the birds acquire and memorize patterns provided by adult models. Many of these birds selectively attend to the songs of their own species. This is similar to human infants who preferentially imitate human sounds rather than others in their environment [8]. Charles Darwin was one of the first to note the similarity between this early stage of song development and human infant babbling.

During the plastic song stage, sound patterns begin to be recognizable as adult in form, but they are still highly variable. As birds progress to the adult or stable song phase, the patterns become stereotyped and are said to have 'crystallized'. Birds learn to produce more song patterns than they will eventually use as an adult. For example, there can be five times the number of song patterns in the plastic than in the stable phase. A similar situation exists in human infants who produce a wider range of sounds than are ultimately used in the language they are acquiring.

Some song birds, such as canaries and red-winged blackbirds, are able to learn new songs throughout their life span, while other species have sensitive periods that are limited to a few days after hatching. For example, learning peaks between 10 and 50 days of age in song sparrows. If these birds are not exposed to song models during this time they develop highly abnormal song.

There may also be critical or sensitive periods of speech/language development in humans. Most of our information on this topic has come from behavioral observations of the learning of second spoken or signed languages (such as American sign language). These and more recent electrophysiological data suggest that age of exposure significantly influences the capacity of humans to acquire language, and in turn, influences the brain organization of the second language system. It is certainly difficult for adult speakers to learn to produce the sounds of a second language correctly, and foreign accents are particularly pronounced if the speaker learns the second language after puberty. Recent data suggest that accent-free pronunciation may require language exposure at a much earlier age, perhaps before 6.

The fact that some song birds renew their song each year has led to some very interesting observations [7]. Stable song lasts for the duration of the breeding season in male canaries. The song then becomes unstable and many new song patterns emerge. This seasonal change in song pattern is associated with dramatic changes in the neural organization of the song control system. There are increases in the volume of both the HVC and RA during the period of song development in the spring and corresponding decreases in these nuclei after the breeding season. The volume changes and seasonal changes in song pattern are in turn related to seasonal fluctuations of testosterone in the male. More complex song patterns and increases in the volumes of HVC and RA occur when female canaries receive intramuscular injections of testosterone. It is interesting to note that there are sex-related differences in the cognitive capabilities of the human brain (including speech and language) that may be due, at least in part, to hormonal influences.

The growth and regression of HVC and RA nuclei appear to be related to the birth and death of neurons, and to changes in dendritic growth and synapse formation, at least within RA. These anatomical changes are thought to represent the neural substrates of the new song motor patterns. It is evident that speech and language also develop in the human infant during a period of growth and maturation of the brain [9]. There has been much conjecture that the establishment of functional connections between the auditory ('Wernicke's') and speech motor ('Broca's') cortical centres coincides with the development of speech and language, but the data to support this hypothesis are lacking.

Non-human primates

Our best models for speech motor control mechanisms may be non-human primates, and for this reason there has been a long standing interest in the language capabilities of these animals. Specifically, people have tried to find out if gorillas and chimpanzees have the capabilities to develop human-like communication. The results of these experiments remain controversial, and it is still not clear that apes possess the capacity for language formation.

What is clear is that non-human primates have much different sound-generating systems than humans. As discussed above, the supraglottal vocal tract gives rise to the acoustic cues needed to differentiate specific speech sounds. In apes, the larynx is located high in the neck, and this configuration brings the epiglottis close to the soft palate. This may allow the lower airway to be more securely closed during swallowing, but it has some negative consequences for speech sound generation. Human infants possess vocal tracts that are very similar to apes, perhaps to maximize the protection of the airway during suckling. It has even been suggested that human infants are able to breathe and swallow at the same time, but this supposition was based on anatomical rather than physiological observations. The available physiological data show that the airway closes during swallowing in human infants and that respiration is interrupted. In fact, a review of the literature reveals that respiration is inhibited prior to swallowing in all species tested including cats, dogs, monkeys and, in our own experiments, rabbits [10]. Nevertheless, the 'ape-like' configuration of the vocal tract appears to limit infants' speech-generating capabilities until the position of the larynx changes during growth to approximate that of the adult.

Neural control

Non-human primates possess complex vocal repertoires that are important for social communication [11]. Many of these natural patterns can be reliably elicited by stimulation of specific brain areas, and these areas appear to be interconnected to form vocal control systems.

Electrical stimulation has been used to show that some calls are represented in the anterior limbic cortex, including orbital, cingulate and temporal cortices. Monkeys can be trained to make conditioned calls and these, but not other parts of the vocal repertoire, are lost after bilateral lesions of limbic cortex. Stimulating the neocortex does not give rise to vocal responses, although stimulation of the lateral face area of the precentral gyrus causes contractions of laryngeal, tongue and facial muscles. In contrast, stimulation of the corresponding region of the cortex in chimpanzees does elicit vocalization.

There are also clear differences between chimpanzees and monkeys in the connections of the motor cortex with laryngeal motoneurons. In chimpanzees, there are direct corticobulbar projections to the nucleus ambiguus (NA) that do not appear to exist in the other non-human primate species. Lesions of the motor and prefrontal cortices, the homologue of Broca's area (which is small in non-human primates) and larger parts of the motor, prefrontal and temporal cortices in macaques apparently have no effect on vocalization, but similar lesions result in profound deficits in humans. These data have been interpreted as evidence of a phylogenetic trend towards greater cortical control over vocalization in primates. Other portions of the forebrain, including parts of the amygdala and hypothalamus, appear to be involved in the control of affective vocalization; that is, vocalization linked to particular emotional states [11]. This suggestion was made because monkey calls evoked by electrical stimulation are often accompanied by other motor and autonomic reactions, similar to those observed during changes in motivational or emotional state.

The anterior limbic cortex appears to have a role in vocalization only in primates. The dorsal cingulate gyrus projects to the hypothalamic, and amygdaloid vocalization areas, as well as the PAG/parabrachial region. In fact, all vocalization areas innervate the PAG/parabrachial region, and in turn, the PAG projects to the NA. Electrical stimulation of the motoneurons in the NA gives rise only to components of the calls; natural sounding vocalizations are not elicited.

Compared with bird song, we know very little about the development of primate vocalization, although the evidence does suggest that most monkey calls are innate. Deafened infant macaque monkeys develop normal call patterns, but comparable data for apes are not available. Monkeys, like some song birds and human infants (and in fact, most animal species who communicate through sound), are most responsive to calls produced by members of their own species.

> ▶ Many of the substrates for speech are present in animals that communicate through sound (e.g. birds and non-human primates).
> ▶ Song birds possess rich and diversified song patterns. Their vocal control systems are hierarchically organized with several areas of the brain involved in song patterning and production. Seasonal changes in song pattern are associated with dramatic hormonally mediated changes in the neural organization of the song control system.
> ▶ Non-human primates possess complex vocal repertoires that are important for social communication. Many of these call patterns can be elicited by stimulation of specific brain sites, and these areas are connected to form vocal control systems. There appears to be a phylogenetic trend towards greater cortical control over vocalization in primates.

Human speech motor control

Cortical mechanisms

Much of what we know about the role of the cortex in speech and language has come from observing the effects of brain damage [9]. Some insight has also been gained from electrical stimulation of brain sites during surgery and from the recording of electroencephalogram (EEG) potentials in normal subjects [9,12]. Brain imaging techniques have only recently been applied to the understanding of speech and language, but most of the studies monitored changes in cortical metabolic rate during the perception of verbal information, as opposed to speech production.

It should be noted that there are sometimes severe limitations in the data gathered with the techniques listed above. Specifying the location and extent of lesions is particularly difficult, and imaging procedures, such as positron emission tomography (PET), that are used to locate areas of increased cortical function suffer from a lack of resolution and a great deal of inter- and intra-subject variability. Despite these limitations, some general principles of the organization for speech production have emerged.

Lateralization of function

A variety of behavioural observations and experimental procedures have revealed that the two cerebral hemispheres possess different cognitive capabilities. In most individuals, the left hemisphere appears to be specialized for linguistic processing and the sequencing of speech movements. The lateralization of function is paralleled by anatomical asymmetries. For example, the lateral sulcus is longer in the left than on the right cerebral hemisphere, and the planum temporale, part of Wernicke's area (Brodmann's area 22, Fig. 6) is larger on the left.

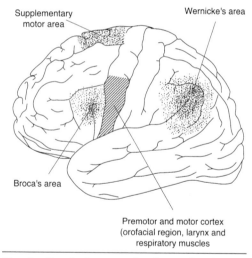

Fig. 6. Cortical control of vocalization in humans

This diagram shows the cortical areas that are known to be important in the patterning of speech and the transmission of the appropriate commands to the lower motor centres. Broca's, Wernicke's and supplementary motor areas are stippled to show that the boundaries and functions of these speech areas are uncertain. The areas of the premotor and motor cortices that control the major groups of motor nerves that are active during speech are more clearly defined (indicated by cross-hatching).

There may also be subcortical lateralization of language function, because portions of the left thalamus appear to be specialized for language and speech motor tasks.

Broca's area

It has been over 130 years since Paul Broca presented his clinical observations of the speech disturbances following lesions of the left frontal cortex. As a result of post-mortem examination of eight patients, Broca suggested that lesions affecting the posterior third of the left third frontal convolution severely disrupted speech output (see Fig. 6). Since that time, this region of the cortex, Broca's area (Brodmann's areas 44 and 45) has been considered to be one of the essential structures controlling speech. Broca's patients had several deficits including difficulty in initiating and sequencing speech sounds, and this 'motor' aphasia carries Broca's name. It is characterized by language that is severely reduced in complexity, and speech may be slowed, effortful and telegraphic; distortions of speech sounds are common. The difficulty that these patients have with the sequencing of speech sounds appears to reflect errors of inter-articulatory coordination. For example, there are differences between patients and normal controls in the timing of voicing relative to consonant articulation. Although these aphasic symptoms were originally linked to lesions of Broca's area, it is now generally accepted that classical Broca's aphasia appears when the damage extends to surrounding areas in the frontal and parietal lobes, and to deeper structures. If the lesions are limited to Broca's area the symptoms are transient.

Apraxia of speech is another clinical entity that may result from damage to Broca's and related cortical areas. This disorder is characterized by problems in the planning and sequencing of speech gestures, without the additional linguistic impairments of Broca's aphasia, like limitations in sentence complexity. Apraxia of speech is considered by some to be a disorder of speech motor programming. However, it should be noted that the existence of apraxia of speech as a clinical entity separate from Broca's aphasia is controversial.

Changes in EEG activity over Broca's area prior to vocalization have been recorded in normal subjects, and cerebral metabolism in that area increases during normal speech, but not during automatic tasks like counting. Electrical stimulation of this area during neurosurgical operations arrests speech production during object naming.

Supplementary motor area

As is the case with other skilled voluntary movements, the supplementary motor area (SMA) is probably involved in the initiation of speech (Fig. 6). In a series of pioneering experiments, Penfield and colleagues explored the effects of localized electrical stimulation of the cerebral cortex in patients being treated for epilepsy and other disorders. When either the right or left SMA was stimulated repetitively, the patients uttered syllables and words with rhythmic changes in pitch and loudness [12].

Recent brain imaging data support the contention that the SMA may be involved in normal speech initiation, and these data are consistent with information from other motor systems. Lesions to the SMA may first result in mutism, followed by severe difficulties in the initiation and production of normal conversational speech, even though the subjects retain the ability to repeat long and complex utterances. The SMA may also play an inhibitory role, as some patients with damage to this area are unable to inhibit unwanted utterances (e.g. swearing).

Motor cortex

The primary motor cortex (MI) is the site of integration of inputs from other cortical and subcortical areas involved in the patterning of speech motor output (Fig. 6). Repetitive stimulation of some sites within the facial sub-division of MI caused some of Penfield's patients to produce continuous vowel sounds that were interrupted at maximum expiration but which began again after inspiration. Cortical blood flow increases over the lateral part of MI during all types of speech, and there are direct projections from MI to hypoglossal, facial, trigeminal and laryngeal motor nuclei in humans. Comparable anatomical data concerning cortical projections to respiratory motoneurons are not available, but magnetic stimulation of the motor cortex in humans has confirmed that there are rapidly conducting cortico-bulbar and cortico-spinal pathways from MI to motor nuclei innervating diaphragm, intercostal, abdominal and other accessory respiratory muscles.

Subcortical mechanisms

Very little is known about subcortical mechanisms involved in speech motor control, although it has long been hypothesized that structures like the thalamus participate in speech and language. Electrical stimulation of various portions of the thalamus during neurosurgical operations has been shown to disrupt speech during object naming tasks.

The cerebellum and basal ganglia must also be important for speech production, because diseases of these structures result in speech disorders [13,14]. For example, lesions to the cerebellum or its connections can cause speech disorders characterized by articulatory inaccuracy and abnormal variations in F_O (impaired prosody). Kinematic and electromyographic (EMG) analyses of peripheral physiological events suggest that cerebellar lesions reduce the velocity and magnitude of speech movements and interfere with the control of movement direction. These findings are consistent with the hypothesis that the cerebellum plays similar roles in the control of limb and speech movements.

The deficits associated with disease also suggest that the basal ganglia and associated structures are important for speech motor control. Parkinson's disease is associated with impairments in prosody, periods of unintelligibility and disordered voice quality [14]. These signs have been attributed to reduced velocity and range of movement and rigidity of the speech musculature. There is some support for the idea that particular speech articulators may be differentially impaired (e.g. lower lip versus upper lip) in some Parkinson's patients. Although limb tremor is a hallmark of the disease, there is no clear evidence that vocal tremor is increased.

Peripheral neural mechanisms

A fundamental question in speech motor control is to what extent, if any, somatosensory and/or auditory feedback interacts with central control signals in the production of speech [15]. The effects of anaesthesia of afferent nerves, and fixation or transient perturbations of articulatory structures, have provided insights into the potential role of sensory feedback in the generation and modification of speech articulatory gestures.

One type of perturbation that has been used frequently to assess the compensatory abilities of the speech production system is the fixation of the jaw by means of a bite-block. Despite large separations of the two jaws, the spectra of vowels are essentially normal when the bite-block is in place. Therefore, the speech motor control system must be capable of developing new articulatory profiles appropriate for the change in jaw position, presumably by modifying the position of the tongue. More recently, attention has been focused on consonants, and it has been shown that bite blocks disturb consonant production, and this leads to significant changes in acoustic, physiological and perceptual measures. Furthermore, there is some improvement in the accuracy of production 10 min after bite-block insertion, suggesting error correction.

Adaptation also occurs during transient perturbations of oral structures. For example, rapid loading of the lower jaw during the production of the sound 'p' is followed by exaggerated movements of the upper and lower lips to bring them together. This is reminiscent of the adaptive capabilities of many other motor systems, and has been used as evidence for the motor equivalence concept discussed above.

Adaptation to perturbations reveals our capacity to use sensory feedback and to form articulatory programs that are appropriate for the changed environment. Sensory feedback may be most important to motor systems during periods of skill acquisition [15]. Hearing is crucial to normal speech sound acquisition, and even minor hearing loss in children can result in errors of speech and language [16]. Information that may be used to control speech production also comes from a variety of sensory receptors located in the respiratory, laryngeal and articulatory systems. The role of auditory and somatosensory inputs in the moment-to-moment corrections of speech gestures in the mature adult system is not clear. However, there is evidence from investigations of the speech of hearing-impaired and aging adults which suggests that certain parameters of speech and/or particular sound classes may require on-line monitoring.

Modification of respiratory reflexes

The demands of speech override the resting respiratory rhythm. This can cause blood gas concentrations to vary significantly from those measured during spontaneous breathing, and there is evidence that some respiratory reflexes are modified during speech. As an example, increasing the $[CO_2]$ of the inspired air causes significantly greater increases in ventilation during spontaneous breathing than when speaking aloud. There is a very rapid shift in the ventilatory response to inspired $[CO_2]$ when changing from spontaneous breathing to speech and vice versa. It has been suggested that the sensitivity of chemostatic respiratory reflexes is lessened to reduce the likelihood of speech being disrupted by changes in respiratory drive. This is one of the pieces of evidence behind the idea that the control of the respiratory system shifts from the brain stem to the cerebral cortex during speech.

However, not all sensory inputs to respiratory motoneurons are suppressed during vocalization. For example, it has been demonstrated that rapid changes in upper airway pressure while subjects sing can elicit short-latency excitatory responses in the intercostal muscles. This reflex may provide active compensation for variations in supraglottal and glottal resistance during speech production.

▶ Several cortical areas may participate in patterning speech. The primary motor cortex (MI) appears to control much of the output through its extensive projections to cranial and spinal motoneurons that innervate the speech musculature. Several cortical areas, including Broca's area and the supplementary motor area, appear to participate in the sequencing and/or initiation of speech sound sequences.

▶ Although relatively little is known about subcortical mechanisms, the cerebellum and basal ganglia are probably important because diseases of these structures result in disordered speech. Subcortical systems may play similar roles in speech and limb movements, because the deficits caused by disease are similar.

Conclusions

▶ In our review, we have attempted to explain how the sounds of speech are generated. We have emphasized that speech is a rapid and dynamic process that demands the simultaneous control of temporally overlapping movements in the respiratory, laryngeal and articulatory systems.

▶ It is apparent that our understanding of the control of these processes is far from complete. However, it does seem that speech, like other skilled human behaviours, is hierarchically controlled and involves several cortical and subcortical structures. In order to learn much more about vocal control in man, we will have to wait for imaging techniques that have high spatial and temporal resolution.

▶ We attempted to separate speech, the motor act, from the higher cognitive processes involved in language comprehension and formation. However, it must be remembered that speech and language are so intimately related that it will always be difficult to determine where language ends and the motor act of speech begins.

We thank Drs. Shari Baum, Christine Weber-Fox and Fred Cody for their contributions to this review, which was supported by the Fonds de la Recherche en Santé du Québec and the Medical Research Council of Canada. Please note that a much more extensive reference list is available upon request from D.H.M.

References
1. Wilkins, J. (1968) An essay towards a real character, and a philosophical language (1668). In English Linguistics 1500–1600: A collection of facsimile reprints (Alston, R.C., ed.), The Scholar Press Ltd., Menston, U.K.
2. Bell, A.M. (1867) Visible Speech: The Science of Universal Alphabetics; or Self-interpreting physiological letters, for the writing of all languages in one alphabet. Simpkin, Marshall & Co., London

3. Hixon, T.J. (1973) Respiratory function in speech. In: Normal Aspects of Speech, Hearing, and Language (Minifie, F.D., Hixon, T.J. and Williams, F., eds.), pp. 73–126, Prentice-Hall, Englewood Cliffs

4. Broad, D.J. (1973) Phonation. in: Normal Aspects of Speech, Hearing, and Language (Minifie, F.D., Hixon, T.J. and Williams, F., eds.), pp. 127–168, Prentice-Hall, Englewood Cliffs

5. Shadle, C.H., Barney, A.M. and Thomas, D.W. (1991) An investigation into the acoustics and aerodynamics of the larynx. In: Vocal Fold Physiology. Acoustic, Perceptual, and Physiological Aspects of Voice Mechanisms (Gauffin, J. and Hammarberg, B., eds.), pp. 73–82, Singular Publishing Group, Inc., San Diego

6. Marler, P. (1991) The instinct for vocal learning: Songbirds. In: Plasticity of Development (Brauth, S.E., Hall, W.S. and Dooling, R.J., eds.), pp. 107–126, MIT Press, Cambridge, MA

7. Nottebohm, F. (1991) Reassessing the mechanisms and origins of vocal learning in birds. Trends Neurosci. 14, 206–211

8. Kuhl, P.J. (1991) Perception, cognition, and the ontogenetic and phylogenetic emergence of human speech. In: Plasticity of Development (Brauth, S.E., Hall, W.S. and Dooling, R.J., eds.), pp. 73–106, MIT Press, Cambridge, MA

9. Whitaker, H.A. (1976) Neurobiology of Language. In: Handbook of Perception, vol. VII: Language and Speech (Carterette, E.C. and Friedman, M.P., eds.), pp. 121–144, Academic Press, New York, NY

10. McFarland, D.H. and Lund, J.P. (1993) An investigation of the coupling between respiration, mastication, and swallowing in the awake rabbit. J. Neurophysiol. 69, 95–108

11. Ploog, D. (1981) Neurobiology of primate audio-vocal behavior. Brain Res. Rev. 3, 35–61

12. Penfield, W. and Welch, K. (1951) The supplementary motor area of the cerebral cortex. A clinical and experimental study. Am. Med. Assoc. Arch. Neurol. Psychiatry 66, 289–317

13. Barlow, S.M. and Farley, G.R. (1989) Neurophysiology of speech. In: Neural Bases of Speech, Hearing, and Language (Kuehn, D.P., Lemme, M.L. and Baumgartner, J.M., eds.), pp. 146–200, College-Hill Press, Boston

14. Darley, F.L., Aronson, A.E. and Brown, J.R. (1975) Motor Speech Disorders. Saunders, Philadelphia

15. Smith, A. (1992) The control of orofacial movements in speech. Crit. Rev. Oral Biol. Med. 3, 233–267

16. Osberger, M.J. and McGarr, N.S. (1982) Speech production characteristics of the hearing impaired. In: Speech and Language: Advances in Basic Research and Practice (Lass, N.J., ed.), pp. 221–283, Academic Press, New York

17. Hirano, M. (1981) Clinical Examination of Voice, Springer-Verlag, New York

6

Impairment of skilled manipulation in patients with lesions of the motor system

Kerry R. Mills

University Department of Clinical Neurology, The Radcliffe Infirmary, Oxford OX2 6HE, U.K.

Introduction

The skilled manipulation of objects, often with both hands simultaneously, is a feature of behaviour which sets humans apart from other primates. This skill can achieve remarkable complexity: a violinist can play a 3-octave scale with one bow movement in about 1 s. This movement requires, with one hand the accurate sequential placement of digits to within 1 mm at regular intervals of 40 ms, and with the other arm a simultaneous constant velocity extension movement of the forearm. The whole movement is accomplished on a background of postural fixation of the head, neck and shoulder on one side to fixate the instrument, but with free movement at the shoulder on the other. The movement will have been practised many times to achieve accuracy, speed and fluidity; at first the player will have used auditory, visual, somatosensory and muscle afferent feedback, i.e. the movement will have been performed in a 'closed-loop' mode. Finally, the movement can be accomplished almost automatically, the speed of finger placements leaving no time for corrections once the sequence has been initiated, i.e. the movement takes place in an 'open-loop' mode. Other more mundane examples of skilled movements, such as doing up a shirt button with one hand and without looking, are performed daily without effort. Here, the skill involves finely directed finger movements continuously guided by sensory feedback. By skilled movements then, we mean movements which require precision and speed and which may be learnt and developed by a process of repetition in the closed-loop mode to become so automatic that open-loop operation is achieved.

Skilled movements are taken for granted by healthy individuals, but when they are even only minimally impaired by disease, great disability can result. Patients with, for example, a small cortical lesion may have no difficulty walking and speaking but may be greatly disabled by their inability to move their fingers accurately as in writing or using a knife and fork.

It is now generally thought that skilled movements, especially of the hand, are dependent on the fastest fibres of the corticospinal tract which make strong monosynaptic connections with motoneurons. Indeed, in infants, the corticospinal tract is unmyelinated and the development of skilled movements appears to occur pari passu with myelination [1].

Patterns of motor impairment

Clinicians have long recognized a number of patterns of motor disturbance in disease. These can be very broadly categorized as: weakness, spasticity, rigidity, ataxia, akinesia and apraxia. It is unusual to find a single type of abnormality in one patient. The distribution of the abnormalities, e.g. single nerve innervation, single limb, bilateral proximal, unilateral upper and lower limb, global, etc. allows the clinician to locate the lesion in the nervous system. The evolution of the motor abnormality over time gives a clue as to the pathology involved. For example, vascular occlusion can lead to immediate paralysis whereas a tumour may produce only slowly progressive symptoms and signs. The clinical term 'upper motoneuron lesion' is frequently encountered and is often used interchangeably with 'pyramidal lesion' or 'corticospinal lesion'. This can lead to confusion since pure pyramidal lesions are very rare if we include in the term only lesions of the medullary pyramids. Lesions at other locations affecting fibres destined to travel in the pyramids invariably affect other fibre systems. Similarly, corticospinal lesions imply a lesion of the corticospinal tract but they also always involve other descending fibre systems. The term upper motor neuron lesion then, although lacking precision, enjoys continued clinical usage and implies a particular constellation of signs — weakness, hyper-reflexia, spasticity and extensor plantar responses. Similarly, the term 'lower motor neuron lesion' refers to any lesion between the spinal motor neuron and the neuromuscular junction.

Muscle weakness

Muscle weakness often arises from disease in the pathway from spinal motoneuron to muscle fibre, often described as lower motoneuron weakness. Thus diseases of the motoneuron itself (e.g. Motor Neuron Disease), lesions of the ventral roots (e.g. cervical radiculopathy), lesions of the motor axons (e.g. peripheral neuropathy), lesions of the neuromuscular junction (e.g. myasthenia gravis) and lesions of the muscle fibre (e.g. muscular dystrophy) all give rise to weakness, often in a characteristic distribution, and often accompanied by wasting of the muscles. Muscle weakness, per se, naturally gives rise to impairment of skilled movements but only in so far as it limits the range of forces to which the central mechanisms have access. A patient with peripheral neuropathy can continue to perform delicate finger movements even when maximum strength is substantially reduced. This ability may, however, be compromised by associated problems with peripheral sensory axons. If motoneuron discharge is recorded from a patient with a lower motoneuron lesion, the firing rate achieved during maximum voluntary contraction is higher than that seen in normal subjects; the central drive to the motoneuron is, it appears, greater in an attempt to compensate for the reduced force output.

A second and quite different type of muscle weakness is caused by lesions of the upper motor tracts. In lesions of the upper motor tracts, movements rather than muscles are affected. The distribution of weakness in a limb is often characteristic in the upper limb affecting flexors more than extensors and in the lower limb extensors more than flexors. Upper motoneuron weakness is often accompanied by spasticity. The lesion causing such signs may lie anywhere from the cortex to the spinal motoneuron. If motoneuron discharge is recorded from a patient with an upper motoneuron lesion, the firing rate achieved during maximal voluntary contraction is lower than that seen in healthy subjects; it appears as if the central drive to the motoneuron has been reduced.

> ▶ Motor disturbance in disease is broadly categorized as weakness, spasticity, rigidity, ataxia, akinesia or apraxia, but patients often have more than one category of abnormality.
> ▶ The distribution of abnormalities allows the clinician to identify the region of the brain affected; the evolution of the abnormalities gives a clue as to the likely pathology.
> ▶ Upper motoneuron lesions often cause weakness, exaggerated tendon reflexes, spasticity and extensor plantar responses.
> ▶ Lower motoneuron lesions cause muscle weakness and often muscle wasting.

Spasticity and rigidity

Muscle 'tone' is a difficult term: clinicians subjectively assess tone by passively moving a limb and estimating the degree of resistance to movement. This passive resistance will include mechanical factors related to the elasticity of joints and tendons as well as the intrinsic resistance of muscle to stretch. Spasticity refers to an increase in resistance to passive stretch of muscle which is velocity dependent, greater resistance being encountered at higher velocities of stretch. Spasticity can vary greatly in severity from the mildest increase in resistance, when, for example, on passively supinating the forearm, the clinician can detect a distinct 'catch'. At the other end of the scale, severely spastic limbs may be held flexed in a continuous state of contraction, any attempt to stretch them leading to alternating reflex contractions of agonist and antagonist muscles, an effect termed clonus. Spasticity is accompanied by exaggeration of deep tendon reflexes. Both phenomena are related to an increase in the excitability of spinal motoneurons which discharge easily when excited by a peripheral input from muscle afferents. The precise mechanism of this increased motoneuron excitability in not completely understood but may well be related to a reduction in tonic inhibition from above either direct to the motoneuron or presynaptically at Ia terminals [2].

Spasticity leads to severe impairment of skilled movements. The increased resistance to movement felt by the examiner of a spastic limb will also be felt by its owner when attempting a voluntary contraction.

Another, and quite different, disturbance of muscle tone is what clinicians refer to as rigidity. Here, the increase in passive resistance is not velocity dependent and the deep tendon reflexes are not exaggerated. On passive movement resistance is encountered over the whole range of movement and in more severe cases may be accompanied by a ratchet-like quality, as if the muscle is stretched in a series of discrete steps, so called cog-wheel rigidity. This form of motor abnormality is often caused by disorders affecting extra-pyramidal central motor pathways and is often accompanied by other symptoms such as tremor and bradykinesia.

Ataxia

Ataxia is an incoordination of movement, manifested by inaccuracies of placement of limbs or defects in the timing or patterning of muscle contractions. Clinicians detect ataxia with such tests as heel–toe walking or finger–nose movements. In its worst form, ataxic patients may be unable to stand or walk because of gross incoordination of the postural musculature. Milder forms of ataxia are manifest as jerkiness of movement or inaccurate placements. Ataxia may be due to either lesions of the cerebellum or its connections, or to gross defects in the sensory inputs from the periphery, so called sensory ataxia. This latter phenomenon emphasizes the importance of sensory feedback in the accomplishment of skilled movements.

Akinesia

This is a disinclination to move or a poverty of movement and is seen in basal ganglia disease. There may also be bradykinesia, a slowness of movement, and a variety of involuntary movements, tremor, chorea or ballismus. Thus patients with Parkinson's disease have difficulties initiating movements, but once they have started to move, execute movements slowly and they may have a tremor of the fingers at about

5–8 Hz, the so-called pill-rolling tremor. Cogwheel rigidity of muscles may also be evident.

Apraxia

This is a disorder of the higher organization of movement and its initiation. Patients with motor apraxia have no weakness, spasticity or reflex change but are unable to perform complex movements which were formerly second nature. For example a patient with motor apraxia when given a toothbrush may be quite unable to illustrate how it would be used. When its use is demonstrated by the examiner, the patient can now copy the movement exactly. The patient appears to be unable to access the particular motor program required. Pure apraxia as described here is rare. Often there are other defects in cognition; one must be sure that the patient has understood the task. Apraxia is one of a larger group of so-called disconnection syndromes in which different cortical areas have become separated by a lesion [3].

> ▶ Spasticity is an increased resistance to passive stretch of a muscle which is velocity dependent.
> ▶ Rigidity is an increased resistance to passive stretch, present over the whole range of movement, not velocity dependent and having a 'ratchet'-like quality.
> ▶ Ataxia is inco-ordinated movement due to defects in the timing and patterning of muscle contractions.
> ▶ Akinesia is disinclination to move often associated with bradykinesia (slowness of movement) and involuntary movements, e.g. tremor.
> ▶ Apraxia is a disturbance of the higher organization of movement resulting in inability to perform complex activities even though there is no weakness, spasticity or ataxia.

Effects of motor tract lesions

The cortical areas concerned with movement in humans are located in the precentral region (primary motor cortex, Brodmann's area 4), in the frontal lobe on the lateral convexity of the hemisphere between the primary motor cortex and the frontal eye fields (premotor cortex) and on the mesial surface of the frontal lobe, above the cingulate gyrus (supplementary motor area). Whereas stimulation of the primary motor cortex produces simple muscle contractions, stimulation of the premotor or supplementary motor areas produces complex movements, often bilateral and involving several joints. The large pyramidal cells of Betz are found in the primary motor cortex but are absent from other motor cortical areas. Both the premotor cortex and the supplementary motor area project to the primary motor cortex but appear to have separate inputs from sensory and visual cortex as well as thalamic nuclei and cerebellum. The premotor cortex and the supplementary motor area are thought to be involved in the temporal patterning of complex movements, especially bimanual tasks. Recently it has been suggested that the premotor cortex is more involved when movement is required in response to an external stimulus whereas the supplementary motor area is concerned more with internally generated movements [4].

Clinical neurology is founded on the correlation of physical signs with known brain lesions to provide the database with which to make diagnoses. The process has built up over many decades and is now improved by imaging techniques such as computed tomography, magnetic resonance imaging and positron emission scanning. Whereas in animals it is possible to make discrete cortical lesions, in patients lesions are rarely circumscribed and almost always involve several cortical areas and variable amounts of subcortical white matter. Even with modern imaging, it may not be possible to assess the full extent of nerve cell impairment since increased pressure, hypoxia or oedema around a lesion may be undetectable. The clinical effects of a motor tract lesion evolve over time; a cortical lesion may initially produce weakness and hypotonia, then weakness with spasticity and eventually only impairment of fine finger movements.

Pure lesions of the primary motor cortex in man are rare; the lesions almost always involve adjacent areas of motor or sensory cortex, or include subcortical white matter as well. The initial effect is a paralysis affecting the particular limb represented by the region of motor cortex affected. Distal muscles are always much more severely affected than proximal ones. Depending on the nature of the

lesion, function may return and the patient may ultimately be left with only a minimal impairment of dexterity and independent finger movements. Spasticity may or may not develop; this seems to depend on the degree to which other motor areas, particularly the supplementary motor area, are also involved.

Unilateral supplementary motor area lesions in man result initially in reduction of spontaneous motor activity on both sides but more pronounced contralateral to the lesion, and an impairment of bimanual skills. The effects may resolve over time to leave a deficit only in rhythmic bimanual finger movements.

Lesions of the premotor area in man appear to cause impairment in the coordination of proximal movements on the two sides, such as pedalling. Independent and bimanual finger movements appear to be preserved and there is little change in muscle tone [5].

Lesions of the parietal cortex may also cause motor disturbance, through disconnection of the sensory input to premotor, supplementary motor and primary motor cortices.

Cutting of both pyramids in monkeys leads to surprisingly few deficits; the animals can still climb and walk. The same is probably also true in man because neurosurgical division of the pyramids, an old strategy for the treatment of involuntary movements, has been documented to cause little defect in coarse movements with discrete finger movements being principally affected. Combined with anatomical data on the increasing numbers and connectivity within motor neuron pools of corticospinal fibres, this has strengthened the idea that the corticospinal tract, especially the fast-conducting component subserves the increasing ability of primates, culminating in man, to move their fingers accurately and independently.

Complete spinal cord lesions in man initially cause a flaccid paralysis of muscles below the segmental level of the lesion and no change to those above. After this initial period of spinal shock, a profound spasticity develops which may ultimately lead to powerful flexion of the legs and painful flexor spasms.

▶ Stimulation of primary motor cortex produces simple muscle contractions, whereas stimulation of premotor or supplementary motor areas produces complex, often bilateral movements.

> ▶ Primary motor cortex lesions in man can produce paralysis in a limb with distal muscles most severely affected.
> ▶ Lesions of the supplementary and premotor areas tend to produce defects in bimanual skills.
> ▶ Complete spinal cord lesions initially produce flaccid paralysis, which evolves into profound spasticity.

Neurophysiological investigation of voluntary movements in man

A number of techniques are available to study, albeit indirectly, the human motor system in action. At the basic level, clinicians have developed tests of skilled movement, such as the 9-hole peg test in which the time taken to insert nine pegs into small holes is recorded. Simple measures of muscle force are also available utilizing hand-held dynamometers or fixed-strain gauges; these have the advantage of directly measuring relevant parameters of function, but give little clue as to the mechanism of any impairment.

Recording of muscle electrical activity
Just as the force output of muscle can be used as an overall measure of output of the motor system, so electromyographic activity can be used to measure the output of spinal motoneurons. Simple surface recordings can be used to determine the timing or patterning of a large number of muscles during complex movements. The finer definition afforded by single motor unit recordings with needle electrodes allows statements to be made about the output of single spinal motoneurons. In healthy subjects low-threshold motor units begin to fire at about 8–10 Hz and their firing rate is modulated upwards during stronger force contractions to a maximum of about 25 Hz. In patients with lower motor neuron lesions, firing rates of the reduced number of motor units in the muscle may reach tonic firing rates of 50–60 Hz. In contrast, if a muscle is affected by an upper motor neuron lesion, then firing rates may remain low at 10–15 Hz, even though the patient is making a maximal effort to activate the muscle. It appears as though the central drive to the motoneurons is reduced.

There is considerable convergence of corticospinal fibres on to single spinal motoneurons. There is also evidence in man, as in other primates, of considerable divergence within motor unit pools of descending motor commands. An estimate of this common drive to motoneurons may be obtained in man by the technique of motor unit train cross-correlation [6]. The timing of the discharge of one motor unit being driven tonically by volition is related to the discharge of a second motor unit either in the same or in a different muscle (Fig. 1). It is found that the discharge of one motor unit occurs, more frequently than expected by chance, close in time to the discharge of the other motor unit; the time course of the cross-correlogram peak suggests that the common drive to the two motoneurons is monosynaptic. This short-term synchrony occurs not only between most motor units of the same muscle, but also to some extent between different muscles of the same limb. Thus motor units in the first dorsal interosseous muscle have their discharges synchronized with motor units in finger adductors and finger extensors, although the strength of synchrony is weaker for more distant muscles. Similarly, when a muscle has multiple functions, e.g. the first dorsal interosseous muscle in the hand participates in finger flexion and extension as well as abduction, the degree of synchronization of its motor units has been shown to be task dependent. The origin of this short-term synchrony is almost certainly central since vibration of the muscle to activate muscle afferents has no effect, but lesions of the corticospinal tract cause it to disappear below the lesion.

The degree of short-term synchronization has been found to vary in certain conditions. In spasticity, for example, it is suggested that the size of common excitatory post-synaptic potentials may be larger than normal.

Bereitschaftspotential
Primate experiments have shown that some motor cortex cells begin to discharge some 100 ms before the onset of a movement trained to occur in response to an external stimulus. In humans, electrical activity can be recorded indirectly from the brain using scalp electrodes. If self-paced finger movements are used to trigger electronic back averaging of cortical activity, a slowly rising potential, variously called the pre-movement potential, readiness potential or

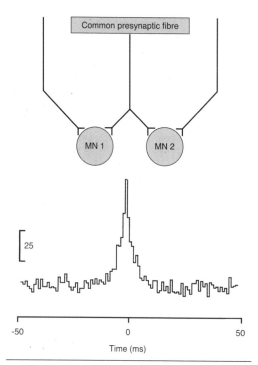

Fig. 1. Divergence of central drive over common presynaptic fibres to different motoneurons

Both shared and unshared descending inputs to a pair of motoneurons (MN1 and MN2) are shown above. Below is a cross-correlogram of the discharges of one MN relative to the discharges of the other at time zero. Both motor units were in the first dorsal interosseous muscle of a healthy subject. The central peak in the cross-correlogram indicates that the motor units tend to discharge in a synchronized fashion more often than would be expected by chance. The shape of the central peak suggests that both MNs are driven by monosynaptic excitatory postsynaptic potentials originating from a common presynaptic fibre.

Bereitschaftspotential, can be recorded over a large area of cortex (Fig. 2). Remarkably, the potential starts some 1 or 1.5 s before the actual execution of the movement; it appears that the intention to move the finger is recordable before the individual is aware that he has made the decision to move. The potential is thought to be produced by two basic cortical generators. The early activity occurring 1.5 to 0.75 s before movement is symmetrical and maximal at the vertex; it probably represents activity in the supplementary motor areas. Later activity is of higher amplitude over the hemisphere contralateral to the movement and is thought to reflect activation of primary motor cortex [7]. This has been used to suggest that supplementary motor area is concerned with initiation and preparation for movement and feeds forward instructions to primary motor cortex for execution. Such time resolution is not possible with blood-flow-imaging techniques which have also been used to investigate cerebral activity before movement onset [8].

Cortical stimulation

The ability to stimulate percutaneously and without pain the central nervous system of awake and co-operative humans has opened up new areas for investigation both in terms of the early diagnosis of neurological disease and the further understanding of normal and abnormal motor control [9]. The magnetic stimulator is an essentially simple device: a brief pulse of electric current is passed through a coil which then generates an intense magnetic field permeating unattenuated into surrounding media. Any electrical conductor, such as the brain, in the vicinity of the coil will have currents induced within it; these induced currents are capable of exciting cerebral neurons. A single weak magnetic stimulus to the scalp probably excites corticospinal tract cells trans-synaptically; stronger stimuli may excite cells directly. The effect of a single stimulus is to cause a high-frequency (500–1000 Hz) burst of impulses to descend in the fastest corticomotoneuronal fibres of the corticospinal tract; the spinal motoneurons are engaged by these impulses and if their excitability is high enough and there is sufficient temporal and spatial summation, then the motoneurons fire, causing a muscle contraction. Intrinsic hand muscles are the most easily excited from brain stimulation but all voluntary muscle, including diaphragm, paraspinal muscle, facial muscle and sphincters appears to be accessible from cortical stimulation. Single scalp shocks probably also bring into play inhibitory mechanisms: if a subject maintains a steady voluntary muscle contraction, the initial excitation caused by the stimulus is followed by a silencing of electromyographic activity. The mechanisms underlying this are still unclear but probably involve inhibition at both cortical and spinal levels. Compound responses from muscle may be recorded with surface electrodes or single

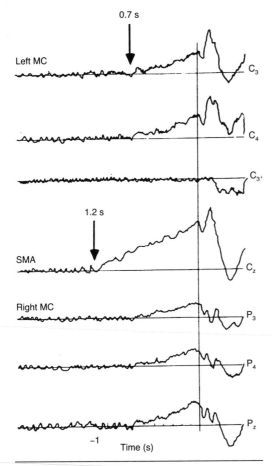

0.7 s

Left MC — C_3

C_4

$C_{3'}$

1.2 s

SMA — C_z

Right MC — P_3

P_4

−1 Time (s) P_z

Fig. 2. Bereitschaftspotential

A left-handed normal subject made 128 self-paced bi-lateral flexion movements of the index fingers and corti-cal activity recorded over the left primary motor cortex (MC) (C_3, C_4), the right primary motor cortex (P_3, P_4) and over the supplementary motor area (SMA) (C_z) was back averaged. The actual movement onset is at time zero. Subscripted letters refer to the International standard convention for scalp electrode placement. Activity over SMA begins 1.2 s before the movement and pre-ceeds activity over primary motor cortex which begins at 0.7 s before the movement. (Reproduced from [7] with permission).

motor unit responses may be recorded with needle electrodes; the former method is used clinically, the latter is useful in research. By subtracting the latency of responses to motor root stimulation from that of cortical stimulation, an estimate of the central motor conduction time may be made.

Magnetic stimuli can cause single motor units to discharge; indeed, the lowest threshold units recruited during a minimal voluntary contraction are the same ones caused to fire by brain stimuli. This suggests operation of the 'size principle' in both situations; the spinal motoneurons react to the descending command whether this is natural or artificial in the same order. The modulation by magnetic scalp stimulation of tonically active single human motor unit discharges gives important insights into the functioning of corticomotoneuronal connections in humans. If, in a normal subject, recordings are made from a single motor unit, reflecting the discharge of a single spinal motoneuron, the recruitment frequency is about 10 Hz. If a series of suprathreshold magnetic stimuli are now given, it is seen that a proportion of stimuli cause the motor unit to discharge at latencies of around 25 ms. It is further seen that discharge latencies are not constant but vary in discrete steps at intervals of about 1.5 ms. These effects are best seen in peri-stimulus time histograms constructed by logging the times of motor unit discharges in relation to stimuli (Fig. 3).

Recordings from pyramidal tract fibres of monkeys show a sequence of waves following single electrical stimuli of sufficient strength to the exposed motor cortex [10]. The first or D-wave is due to direct excitation of pyramidal tract cells whereas later waves, I-waves, are due to re-excitation of the same pyramidal tract cells by intra-cortical circuits. This descending train of impulses impinge on spinal motoneurons to produce a composite excitatory post-synaptic potential (EPSP) which can be recorded intracellularly [11]. The intervals between D- and I-waves and between subsequent I-waves, and between the components of the composite EPSP are 1–2 ms. By analogy with these findings, the discrete discharge latencies of human motoneurons from scalp stimulation are thought to represent the motoneuron being raised to threshold by one of the separate components of the EPSP [12].

In patients with multiple sclerosis, a condition in which demyelination of central fibres takes place, the peaks of excitation following scalp stimuli may be greatly delayed, occurring some 20 ms later than expected; this is probably due to a reduced conduction velocity in corticomotoneuronal fibres consequent upon fibre demyelination. Delay in the arrival of the motor command at the motoneuron would not

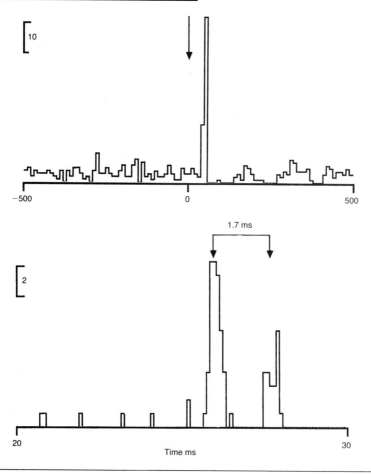

Fig. 3. Cortical stimulation modulates single motor unit discharges
Peri-stimulus time histogram of the discharges of a tonically active single motor unit in first dorsal interosseous muscle of a healthy subject. The times of motor unit discharge, relative to the magnetic stimulus at time zero (arrow), have been logged into bins of width 5 ms. A sharp rise in firing probability (upper Figure) is seen at 25–30 ms after the stimulus. At higher time resolution (0.2 ms binwidth) (lower Figure), the rise in firing probability consists of two distinct subpeaks at an intermodal interval of 1.7 ms. These subpeaks probably reflect two components of the composite excitatory post-synaptic potential induced by repetitive firing of corticomotoneuronal fibres.

necessarily lead to impairment of motor function. However, the phase of excitation is also often dispersed, increasing temporal dispersion at the motoneuron and possibly resulting in its failure to fire with the usual descending command. In some patients, the intervals between histogram peaks may be prolonged, suggesting a frequency-dependent block in the corticospinal volley which may also impair the ability of the motoneuron to reach threshold. Finally, in a few patients, stimulation of the brain may have the effect of suppressing tonic motor unit discharge. One can speculate that in a patient wanting to move the finger, the motor command would instead switch off the motoneurons. Thus study of the corticospinal influence to single spinal motoneurons can suggest mechanisms at the synaptic level which might give rise to weakness and impairment of finger movements in patients.

Central conduction abnormalities (delayed or small-amplitude surface-recorded responses) correlate poorly with neurological signs. A patient may have weakness of an intrinsic hand muscle but not show delayed responses to brain stimulation. Conversely, and of greater clinical importance for early diagnosis, is the finding in about 10% of cases of multiple sclerosis that central motor conduction may be abnormal even when no clinical abnormality can be detected.

▶ Evidence of the divergent monosynaptic corticospinal projection to motoneurons can be obtained by cross-correlation analysis of motor unit discharge, which shows short-term synchronization.
▶ Cortical potentials can be recorded over the supplementary motor area 1.5 s before a self-paced movement and precede potentials over the primary motor cortex.
▶ Magnetic stimulation of the brain can activate the corticospinal projections to motoneurons, single stimuli producing multiple descending volleys.

Conclusions

▶ Study of the derangements in motor control that can result from disease can also teach us about the mechanisms that normally operate.
▶ Estimation of short-term synchronization among motor units of the same and nearby motoneuron pools has confirmed that even simple motor commands are widely distributed in the spinal cord.
▶ Cortical potentials can be recorded up to 2 s before a self-paced movement; activity over the supplementary motor area preceeds that from primary motor cortex.
▶ The finding from brain stimulation that many human muscles, but especially intrinsic hand muscles, have powerful and direct monosynaptic contacts from the motor cortex has highlighted the importance of the fastest fibres of the corticospinal tract in skilled hand movements.

References

1. Eyre, J.A., Miller, S. and Ramesh, V. (1991) Constancy of central conduction delays during development in man: investigation of motor and somatosensory pathways. J. Physiol. **434**, 441–452
2. Rothwell, J.C. (1987) Control of Human Voluntary Movement. Croon Helm, London and Sidney
3. Geschwind, N. (1965) Disconnexion syndromes in animals and man. Part II. Brain **88**, 585–644
4. Passingham, R.E. (1987) Motor Areas of the Cerebral Cortex. Ciba Symp. **132**, pp. 151–164, John Wiley, Chichester
5. Halsband, U., Ito, N., Tanji, J. and Freund, H.-J. (1993) The role of premotor cortex and the supplementary motor area in the temporal control of movement in man. Brain **116**, 243–266
6. Datta, A.K. and Stephens, J.A. (1990) Synchronization of motor unit activity during voluntary contraction in man J. Physiol. (London) **422**, 397–419
7. Kristeva, R. and Deecke, L. (1980) in Motivation, motor and sensory processes of the brain: Electrical potentials, behaviour and clinical use. In: Progress in Brain Research (Kornhuber, H.H. and Deecke, L., eds.), 748–754, Elsevier, Amsterdam
8. Roland, P.E. (1987) Motor Areas of the Cerebral Cortex. Ciba Symp. **132**, 251–268
9. Day, B.L., Dressler, D., Maertens de Noordhout, A., Marsden, C.D., Nakashima, K., Rothwell, J.C. and Thompson, P.D. (1989) Electric and magnetic stimulation of human motor cortex: EMG and single motor unit studies. J. Physiol. (London) **412**, 449–473
10. Porter, R. and Lemon. R. (1993) Corticospinal function in voluntary movements. Monographs of the Physiology Society No. 45, Clarendon Press, Oxford
11. Kernell, D. and Wu, C.-P. (1967) Post-synaptic effects of cortical stimulation on forelimb motor neurones in the baboon. J. Physiol. (London) **191**, 673–690
12. Mills, K.R. (1991) Magnetic brain stimulation: a tool to explore the action of the motor cortex on single human spinal motoneurones. Trends Neurosci. **14**, 401–405

Glossary

Afferent fibres
They transmit impulses from peripheral receptors (in muscles, joints, skin, etc.) to the spinal cord. Different types of afferent fibres can be distinguished which transmit impulses from different types of receptors. These fibres are classified according to their conduction velocity which is related to the thickness of the fibre.

Akinesia
A disinclination to move or difficulty in initiating movement, often associated with bradykinesia (slowness of movement), or involuntary movements such as tremor.

Apraxia
A disturbance of the higher organization of movement such that a patient without weakness, spasticity, etc. is nevertheless unable to perform a complex series of movements, e.g. dressing.

Apraxia of speech
A speech disorder resulting from damage to Broca's and related cortical areas. Characterized by problems in the planning and sequencing of speech gestures, without the additional linguistic impairments of Broca's aphasia.

Articulatory system
Refers to the supralaryngeal vocal tract (e.g. pharynx, soft palate, jaws, lips, and tongue).

Association areas (of cerebral cortex)
Regions of the cerebral cortex which are neither primary sensory (receiving) areas nor primary motor areas and which are believed to be concerned with complex behavioural processes.

Ataxia
An incoordination of movement due to faulty timing or patterning of muscle contractions. It may be due to lesions of the cerebellum or its connections or to diminished peripheral sensory feedback.

Ballism
Sudden, erratic, flinging movements of the limbs following lesions of the subthalamic nucleus.

Ballistic movement
A voluntary movement made as rapidly as possible. The duration of movement (200 ms or less) is too short for any voluntary corrections to be made and the movement is preprogrammed.

Bernoulli forces
Pressure between the vocal folds is inversely proportional to the velocity airflow. Elastic recoil of the stretched vocal fold tissue and Bernoulli forces return the folds to their closed position during each vibratory cycle.

Bereitschaftspotential
A potential recorded over the scalp, with a widespread distribution, in the period 1–1.5 s before a self-initiated voluntary movement.

Broca's aphasia
Motor aphasia involving damage to Broca's area and surrounding areas. Patients may have language that is severely reduced in complexity, and speech may be slowed, effortful, and telegraphic. Distortions of speech sounds are common.

Broca's area
Left frontal cortex (Brodmann's areas 44 and 45) thought to be involved in speech production. Damage to this and surrounding areas may give rise to Broca's aphasia.

Brodmann's areas
A numerical system of subdivisions of the cerebral cortex devised by the histologist Brodmann which is based on cortical cytoarchitecture, e.g. thickness of cortical layering. Over 50 such regions were identified in the human brain with a smaller number in monkeys. Area 1 is the primary somatosensory cortex and area 4 the primary motor cortex.

Caudate
One of the nuclei of the basal ganglia. Together with a second nucleus, the putamen, forms the neostriatum.

Chorea
Involuntary, irregular movements affecting all parts of the body which may produce a dance-like motion (St. Vitus' dance). Probably caused by lesions to the striatum of the basal ganglia. Found in Huntington's disease.

Cingulate motor areas
Motor areas of the cingulate gyrus with corticospinal projections and which give rise to movement when stimulated.

Climbing fibre
Excitatory input fibres to the cerebellum which originate in the inferior olivary nucleus of the medulla. Each climbing fibre contacts 1–10 Purkinje cells in the cerebellar cortex while each Purkinje cells receives an input from a single climbing fibre. Activation of Purkinje cells by climbing fibres produces a powerful response, comprising a high frequency burst of action potentials, known as a complex spike.

Co-articulation
A term used to describe the overlap in time of the articulatory features of different speech sounds.

Conditioned stimulus
A type of stimulus used in the experimental paradigm of classical conditioning as employed by Pavlov at the turn of the century. The essence of the method is the pairing of two stimuli, an unconditioned stimulus (US) and conditioned stimulus (CS). The US, e.g. food or a shock to the leg, always produces an overt response on its own. The CS, e.g. a light or tone, produces either no response or a very weak one. When the CS is repeatedly followed by the US the CS begins to elicit responses as it acts as an anticipatory signal for the US.

Corollary discharge
A neural replica of a motor command signal which may pass to sensory centres and allow evaluation of the afferent input produced by the accompanying movement.

Corpus callosum
A large band of nerve fibres that crosses between and interconnects the cerebral hemispheres.

Cortico-motoneuronal (CM) cell
A corticospinal cell which makes a direct, monosynaptic projection to spinal motoneurons.

Corticospinal projections
Descending projections arising in the frontal and parietal cortical areas and projecting to the spinal cord.

Diplopia
Double vision as, for example, when the two eyes are misaligned.

Direct pathway
A term often applied to one of two main routes (versus indirect pathway) linking the striatum to the internal globus pallidus of the basal ganglia. This route comprises a direct connection between these nuclei.

Dopamine
A common neurotransmitter in the central nervous system. Chemically a catecholamine. Degeneration of dopaminergic neurons of the substantia nigra is believed to cause Parkinson's disease.

Dystonia
A rare disorder characterized by abnormal co-contraction of antagonist muscles which may produce fixed, twisted postures. Associated with disease of the basal ganglia.

Exafference
Sensory input arising from receptor stimulation which is not generated by the body itself, i.e. other than by the body's own movements.

Feedforward control
A form of control system in which the command signal passes directly to the actuator and which does not utilize feedback information about the outcome. Also known as open-loop control. An example is a preprogrammed, ballistic movement whose accuracy depends on the precision of the initial motor command.

Formant frequencies
The resonant modes of the vocal tract filter. The voicing spectrum is modified as it passes through the filter.

Frontal eye fields
A cerebral cortical region (Brodmann's area 8) in front of the primary motor cortex and premotor cortex involved in controlling eye movements.

Functional synergists
Groups of muscles which act together to produce a particular movement.

Fundamental frequency (F_O)
The rate at which the vocal folds open and close. The perceptual correlate of F_O is pitch.

Globus pallidus
A nucleus of the basal ganglia. Divided into internal (medial) and external (lateral) parts,

projecting to the thalamus and subthalamic nucleus, respectively.

Golgi tendon organ (GTO)
The tension receptor of skeletal muscle which consists of several tendon fascicles within a capsule. GTOs are located near the origin of the tendon in series with the muscle. The receptor is more sensitive to active than passive tension and is strongly excited by contraction of the muscle fibres which are attached to its capsule. The signals of GTOs are transmitted by group-Ib afferent fibres to the spinal cord.

Granule cell
A very numerous type of neuron in the deepest 'granular' layer of the cerebellar cortex. They receive, via mossy fibres, a major part of the external input to the cerebellar cortex. The axons of granule cells ascend to the superficial 'molecular' layer. Here they divide in a T-junction to form parallel fibres which make excitatory synapses with the dendritic trees of Purkinje cells in which they produce 'simple spikes'.

Group-Ia fibres
Afferent nerve fibres from the primary (annulospiral) sensory endings of muscle spindle receptors.

Group-Ib fibres
Afferent nerve fibres from Golgi tendon organ receptors.

Group-II fibres
Afferent nerve fibres from (amongst others) the secondary (flowerspray) sensory endings of muscle spindle receptors.

H-reflex (Hoffmann reflex)
The monosynaptic spinal reflex which can be elicited in humans by electrical stimulation of group-Ia afferent fibres (from muscle spindles) within the peripheral nerves. The electrically evoked analogue of the tendon jerk or stretch reflex. H-reflex responses can be recorded by electromyography over the muscle from which the stimulated afferent fibres originate.

Huntington's disease
An inherited disease of the basal ganglia characterized by chorea and progressive mental decline.

Indirect pathway
A term often applied to one of two main routes (versus direct pathway) linking the striatum to the internal globus pallidus of the basal ganglia. This route comprises relays in the external globus pallidus and subthalamic nucleus.

Inferior olive
A nucleus in the medulla whose neurons have axons termed climbing fibres which provide a major source of input to the cerebellum and evoke 'complex spikes' in cerebellar Purkinje cells.

Load receptor
The load receptor of skeletal muscle is the Golgi tendon organ.

Long-latency (polysynaptic or M2) reflex
A reflex, whose reflex arc, in addition to the afferent and efferent neuron, comprises one or more interneurons and, therefore, several synapses in the central nervous system.

Long-term depression (LTD)
A reduction in the activity of a neuron, occurring over a period of hours or days, evoked by an excitatory input due to a decrease in synaptic efficacy.

Long-term potentiation (LTP)
An increase in the activity of a neuron, occurring over a period of hours or days, evoked by an excitatory input due to an enhancement of synaptic efficacy. LTP and LTD are believed to form the basis of learning.

Lower motoneuron lesion
A lesion of the motor pathway between the spinal motoneuron and neuromuscular junction, usually associated with weakness and wasting of muscles.

Magnocellular
Refers to large cells. For instance, the sub-population of large retinal ganglion cells are termed magnocellular neurons.

Metasystem
A supervisor system which operates in parallel with other circuits and acts to automate, calibrate and optimize them.

Mossy fibre
A major source of input to the cerebellum arising from all main sensory systems and from all main motor pathways. These axons end in the granular layer of the cerebellar cortex. A single mossy fibre may contact 400 granule cells as well as Golgi cells.

Motor equivalence
Principle that many muscle activation patterns or movement trajectories can be used to achieve a given movement goal.

MPTP
N-Methyl-4-phenyl-1,2,3,6-tetrahydropyridine. A neurotoxin with specificity for dopaminergic (and noradrenergic) neurons. Produces signs similar to those of Parkinson's disease.

Muscle field
The group of muscles whose activity is facilitated by a single neuron.

Muscle spindle
The length and stretch receptor of skeletal muscle. These receptors consist of bundles of small, specialized, spindle-shaped intrafusal muscle fibres. Muscle spindles are located in parallel with the larger extrafusal fibres. Two main types of afferent nerve fibres supply muscle spindles; one (group Ia) is more sensitive to a change in muscle length (dynamic behaviour) and one (group II) is more sensitive to the absolute length of the muscle (static behaviour). The responsiveness of the receptors depends on the degree of contraction of the intrafusal muscle fibres which is regulated by their motor innervation by gamma motoneurons.

Negative feedback control
A type of control mechanism which compares signals of the output of the system (e.g. movement) with the command signal and uses the resulting difference, termed error signal, to regulate the output. Also known as closed-loop control. Servomechanisms and regulators are examples of feedback control systems designed to produce, respectively, varying and constant outputs.

Parkinson's disease
A common human disease of the basal ganglia involving degeneration of the dopaminergic neurons of the substantia nigra. Patients show tremor, akinesia/bradykinesia and rigidity.

Parvocellular
Refers to small cells. For instance, the sub-population of small retinal ganglion cells are termed parvocellular neurons.

Pitch
The perceptual correlate of the fundamental frequency of vocal fold vibration.

Prefrontal cortex
An association area of cerebral cortex which has a motor function. Located in front of the primary motor and premotor areas. Believed to be involved in selecting strategies of movement according to appropriate cues.

Premotor cortex
A distinct cortical area which, in primates, lies immediately in front of the primary motor cortex.

Presynaptic inhibition
A mechanism, involving an axo-axonic synapse, that results in a decrease in the amount of transmitter released at an excitatory synaptic terminal so that the postsynaptic potential is reduced in size.

Pretectal area
An important visual reflex centre just rostral to the superior colliculus. Mediates the pupillary light reflex, i.e. constriction of the pupil when a light is shone into the eye.

Prosodic elements
Suprasegmental aspects of language such as intonation, stress and rhythm.

Purkinje cell
The output neurons of the cerebellar cortex. These neurons project to the cerebellar nuclei where they exert an inhibitory action.

Pursuit eye movement
Eye movement whose function is to match movements of the fovea of the retina with those of a visual target to ensure clear vision.

Putamen
One of the nuclei of the basal ganglia. Together with a second nucleus, the caudate, forms the neostriatum.

Pyramidal tract
The bundle of descending fibres, all derived from the cerebral cortex, that pass on

the ventral side of the medulla oblongata in the brainstem. In cross-section, the tract has a pyramidal form. Only a proportion of the fibres reach the spinal cord.

Reafference
Sensory input, mainly supplied by proprioceptors, which results entirely from an animal's own movements.

Relatively independent finger movements (RIFM)
Term used to describe those movements which occur when the digits are employed in tasks of high precision, e.g. doing up a button, or retrieving small objects using opposition between the tips of the thumb and index finger.

Retinal ganglion cell
The output neurons of the retina of the eye. The axons of these cells form the optic nerve which transmits visual signals to the brain.

Rigidity
A change in muscle tone manifest as increased resistance to passive stretch, present over the whole range of movement, not being stretch velocity dependent and having a distinctive 'ratchet'-like quality.

Rubrospinal, reticulospinal and vestibulospinal tracts
Descending motor pathways to the spinal cord originating in the red nucleus, reticular formation and vestibular nuclei, respectively.

Saccade
Rapid 'flicking' movements of the eyes which allow new

parts of the visual world to be quickly viewed.

Sensorimotor cortex
The primary somatosensory and motor areas. In the primate these refer to Brodmann's areas 3, 1, 2 and 4, respectively.

Spasticity
A change in muscle tone manifest as an increased resistance to passive stretch which is greater with increasing velocity of stretch. It is usually associated with exaggerated tendon reflexes.

Spike-triggered averaging (STA)
A means of discovering the influence of a single, spontaneously active neuron upon a postsynaptic element or elements. A CM connection between a cortical neuron and the motoneurons of a given muscle can be identified by making an STA of the electromyographic (EMG) activity of the muscles using the spike events of the neuron as triggers for the average. If an excitatory connection exists, post-spike facilitation of the EMG will be evident as a transient peak in the STA.

Striosomes
Groups of densely packed neurons in the striatum of the basal ganglia. Form a sub-population with different biochemical properties and connections from the remainder of striatal neurons (the less densely packed matrix).

Stops
Sounds produced when airflow is rapidly impounded and released.

Stretch reflex
The contraction of a skeletal muscle which results from stretching of the muscle. The best known example is the tendon jerk which is a simple spinal reflex. It is produced by the excitatory action of muscle spindle afferents, stimulated by a brief muscle stretch caused by a tendon tap, upon motoneurons. More prolonged stretch produces later 'long-latency' components thought to be mediated via transcortical pathways.

Stretch receptor
The stretch receptor of skeletal muscle is the muscle spindle.

Subglottal pressure
The pressure generated below the adducted vocal folds by respiratory drive.

Substantia nigra
A nucleus of the basal ganglia located in the midbrain whose cells are packed with melanin. Divided into two parts, pars compacta and pars reticulata, with separate connections to other brain regions.

Subthalamic nucleus
A nucleus of the basal ganglia located in the midbrain beneath the thalamus. Lesions produce ballism/hemiballismus.

Supplementary motor area (SMA)
A cortical motor area lying in the medial wall of the hemisphere.

Transcranial magnetic stimulation (TMS)
Activation of the cortex by electric currents induced by applying a brief but powerful magnetic field over the head using a coil.

Tremor
Involuntary, high frequency, oscillating movements of a limb which produce shaking. There are many forms of tremor of which some occur in health (physiological tremor) and others in disease (e.g. Parkinson's disease, cerebellar disease). The different forms are distinguished by different amplitudes and frequencies and whether they occur at rest or during voluntary movements.

Unconditioned stimulus
A type of stimulus used in the experimental paradigm of classical conditioning as employed by Pavlov at the turn of the century. The essence of the method is the pairing of two stimuli, an unconditioned stimulus (US) and conditioned stimulus (CS). The US, e.g. food or a shock to the leg, always produces an overt response on its own. The CS, e.g. a light or tone, produces either no response or a very weak one. When the CS is repeatedly followed by the US the CS begins to elicit responses as it acts as an anticipatory signal for the US.

Upper motoneuron lesion
A lesion of the upper motor tracts associated with a particular constellation of physical signs including weakness, spasticity, exaggerated deep tendon reflexes and extensor plantar responses.

Vestibulo-ocular reflex (VOR)
A reflex movement of the eyes in response to stimulation of the vestibular apparatus. For instance, the movements of the eyes which occur in the opposite direction to head movements and allow clear vision of visual objects to be retained.

Visual cortex
The primary visual cortex (V1, Brodmann's area 17), also termed the striate cortex because of a prominent stripe of white matter, receives inputs from the lateral geniculate nucleus via the optic radiation. Projections from V1 pass to areas concerned with higher level processing including the prestriate cortex (V2, V3 and V4, Brodmann's area 18 and 19) and thence to the inferotemporal cortex (Brodmann's areas 20 and 21).

Voiced or unvoiced sounds
The distinction being the presence (voiced) or absence (unvoiced) of vocal fold vibration. All English vowels and some consonants (e.g. d) are voiced, while the remaining consonant sounds are unvoiced.

Voicing spectrum
The sound spectrum created by the complex vibration of the vocal folds. Contains the F_O and higher-order harmonics with significant energy up to about 4500 Hz.

Wernicke's area
Left temperoparietal area involved in language formation.

Index

Coventry University